Hospital-Acquired Infections in Intensive Care Unit and their Management

Raja Chakraverty • Asim Kumar Kundu

Hospital-Acquired Infections in Intensive Care Unit and their Management

The Indian Perspective

Springer

Raja Chakraverty
Department of Critical Care Medicine
IPGMER-SSKM Hospital
Kolkata, West Bengal, India

Asim Kumar Kundu
Department of Critical Care Medicine
IPGMER-SSKM Hospital
Kolkata, West Bengal, India

ISBN 978-981-96-0017-5 ISBN 978-981-96-0018-2 (eBook)
https://doi.org/10.1007/978-981-96-0018-2

This Springer imprint is published by the registered company Springer Nature Singapore Pte Ltd.
The registered company address is: 152 Beach Road, #21-01/04 Gateway East, Singapore 189721, Singapore

Dedicated to the loving memory of my father, a professor, writer, and passionate researcher like none before, who always encouraged me to chase my dreams and someone, who like many others, unfortunately lost his life fighting hospital-acquired infections in the intensive care unit.
Miss you a lot

—Raja Chakraverty

Foreword

While most books on critical care and infection control practices place a strong clinical emphasis, which is essential for training future doctors, pharmacists, and nurses working in hospitals and health care facilities, they often do a disservice to future researchers by neglecting their needs. Now, hospital-acquired infections, also known as nosocomial infections, constitute a common, often fatal, and major challenge to the public health infrastructure of any nation, particularly in LMICs like India. Owing to it, health care providers must also be sufficiently equipped to assimilate and interpret the recent grades of evidence of infection prevention, mitigation, and management from laboratory to bedside. This is where this book aims to address the gap.

This book from Springer Nature is timely and addresses antimicrobial resistance in a clear and contextual manner, as well as infection prevention in intensive care units of health care facilities, based on current national and international guidelines. It will stand the test of time and prove to be an indispensable resource for intensivists, surgeons, clinicians, nurses, pharmacists, and researchers working in intensive care, with the common goal of tilting odds in favor of the patient against the backdrop of complex organ dysfunctions and insidious diseases.

Finally, I would like to commend the authors and the reputable publishers for their foresight, vision, and timely publication of this much-needed book.

ICMR-NIRBI
Kolkata, India

Debjit Chakraborty

Preface

Writing a credible book is always a monumental challenge and a great responsibility. With this very important title, we have tried taking up the enormous challenge head-on. This current treatise has been comprehensively curated for all types of medical professionals and students dealing with drugs and infections in intensive care units. It provides an overview of the prevention and management mechanisms for various infections, including catheter associated UTI (CA-UTI), central line-associated bloodstream infections (CLABSI), surgical site infections (SSI), ventilator-associated pneumonia (VAP), hospital-acquired pneumonia (HAP), community-acquired pneumonia (CAP), bedsores of various grades, and *C. difficile* infections. The text aims to present these complex topics in a clear and concise manner, enabling readers to grasp the fundamental principles of infection prevention and management in intensive care units. This book aims to explain various observations and experiments in infection prevention and control, such as hand hygiene and disinfection, that are backed by high-grade evidence, with a focus on better practices and their practical applications in the healthcare industry. Sepsis and multiple organ dysfunction syndrome (MODS) have been taken up elaborately by the authors, which will seamlessly facilitate clarity and understanding in these intricate areas of critical care as per the latest guidelines. This textbook is written for you: students, young faculty members, clinical practitioners, and future researchers. Our beacon of hope rests with all of you. We will be happy to receive your constructive feedback regarding this, which will help us improve our work in subsequent editions.

We extend our heartfelt gratitude to the team of editors and staff at Springer Nature for their untiring efforts in pursuit of excellence and for all their patience and constant encouragement.

Happy Reading everyone!

Kolkata, West Bengal, India

Raja Chakraverty
Asim Kumar Kundu

Contents

Chapter 1
Introduction to Nosocomial Infection

1.1 Introduction

Nosocomial infections present themselves as one of the most intricate challenges to address within the confines of a hospital environment. The onus of hospital-acquired infections (HAI) exerts a significant impact on the financial expenses incurred by patients for medical treatment, thereby exerting a substantial influence on the economic landscape of a developing nation such as India. The indiscriminate use of antibiotics in treating these infections has precipitated the emergence of resistance among microbial agents, while additional complicating factors further exacerbate the scenario. A considerable proportion of HAI cases can be averted by adhering to a range of protocols, which, when coupled with prudent antibiotic administration, can ameliorate the gravity of the issue. Systematic infection control strategies, well-trained hospital personnel, and ongoing monitoring of HAI within healthcare facilities are instrumental in addressing nosocomial infections. Although the capacity to address HAI in a patient can potentially determine their survival post acquiring such an infection, prevention consistently emerges as the most favorable recourse. The reduction of nosocomial infection burdens assumes paramount significance as it substantially influences the overall allocation of resources within both the hospital setting and the nation at large. The incorporation of nanoparticles and nanotechnology for targeted drug delivery holds promise in mitigating antibiotic resistance. By taking cognizance of reports detailing the patterns of nosocomial infections across various medical centers in India, the gravity and repercussions of HAI are brought to light.

Nosocomial infections, also known as hospital-acquired infections (HAI), are infections that manifest within a period of 48 h following admission to a healthcare facility, within 3 days subsequent to discharge, or postoperatively within a span of 1 month according to existing literature [1]. It is imperative that the infection is not in an active state or in the incubation phase during the patient's admission; essentially,

R. Chakraverty, A. K. Kundu, *Hospital-Acquired Infections in Intensive Care Unit and their Management*, https://doi.org/10.1007/978-981-96-0018-2_1

these infections must be acquired through contact with healthcare services as emphasized in various sources [1, 2]. Statistics indicate that approximately 10–20% of patients who are admitted to healthcare facilities in India end up acquiring nosocomial infections during their hospital stay [3]. Notably, intensive care units (ICUs) have been identified as the primary locus for the occurrence of HAI, accounting for a significant quarter of all infections contracted within hospital settings [4]. Within clinical environments, it has been observed that *Staphylococcus aureus* stands out as the most prevalent causative agent of nosocomial infections [5]. Contributing factors to the prevalence of such infections include substandard hygiene practices and conditions, alongside the burgeoning patient population within hospital premises, which collectively exacerbate the situation [6]. Furthermore, the indiscriminate use of non-susceptible antibiotics in the treatment of bacterial infections without prior susceptibility testing represents a critical juncture where the selective proliferation of resistant bacteria due to acquired mutations is highly likely to occur, as underscored in the medical literature [5]. The gravity of the disease itself coupled with the repetitive exposure to various treatment modalities among patients admitted to ICUs establishes a fertile ground for recurrent infections within this particular patient cohort [7]. Research findings point toward the nosocomial transmission of neonatal infections as a significant contributor to neonatal mortality rates in India, ultimately fostering the emergence of more strains of antimicrobial-resistant bacteria [8]. In considering the source of infection, it is noted that it can either be endogenous or exogenous in nature, with the latter being more predominant in occurrence according to prevailing data. Vulnerable demographic groups such as the elderly and immunocompromised individuals, including those with diabetes as well as patients with drainage devices and intubation, are particularly susceptible to contracting nosocomial infections within healthcare settings [4, 6].

Ventilator-associated pneumonia (VAP), intravenous line-associated bloodstream infections (BSI), and catheter-related urinary tract infection (UTI) persist as common healthcare-associated infections (HAI) within medical facilities. Factors such as prolonged surgical procedures, inadequate nutritional intake, cardiac cachexia, and hypothermia contribute to the occurrence of these infections, subsequently elevating the overall management expenses and amplifying the mortality rates. According to the National Nosocomial Infections Surveillance System (NNIS), surgical site infections (SSI) rank as the third most frequently documented HAI in India. Interestingly, even nonpathogenic microorganisms can lead to HAI in individuals with compromised immune systems. Nosocomial infections manifest either as sporadic outbreaks or as endemic occurrences within healthcare facilities. It is noteworthy to acknowledge that infections contracted by healthcare personnel are classified as nosocomial. Although intensive care units (ICUs) typically constitute less than 10% of total bed occupancy in most hospitals, a substantial 20% of nosocomial infections transpire in these critical care settings [9]. The incidence and prevalence of nosocomial infections, alongside the levels of microbial resistance, exhibit significant variations based on geographical location and distinct ICU environments. The burden of HAI is notably heavier on low- and middle-income countries in terms of healthcare expenditure. The research underscores that HAI resulting in prolonged ICU stays are linked to a twofold escalation in treatment costs. Alarmingly, statistics reveal that 15 out of every 100 hospitalized patients contract at least one nosocomial infection, with a mortality rate of one in every 10 infected individuals [10–16]. This trend is largely attributed to the necessity of potent antibiotics to combat multidrug-resistant pathogens, leading to extended hospitalizations and increased diagnostic procedures. A substantial 23.6% of overall mortality is directly linked to HAI, underscoring the critical impact of these infections on patient outcomes. It is imperative to recognize that complete eradication of HAI is unattainable; hence, the optimal approach lies in stringent preventive strategies, early detection protocols, and efficient control measures to mitigate transmission within healthcare settings.

1.2 Literature Review

A comprehensive literature review was undertaken to thoroughly examine the data concerning nosocomial infections and its implications in the context of healthcare facilities in India. The researchers conducted searches on various electronic databases such as PubMed, MEDLINE, Embase, and Google Scholar, utilizing a specific set of keywords and their combinations, including nosocomial infections, hospital-acquired infections, COVID-19, medical ICU, and antibiotics. The search strategy covered articles published over a substantial timeframe from 1993 to 2023, to capture a wide range of relevant literature on the subject. Furthermore, beyond electronic database inquiries, the researchers manually screened the reference lists of pertinent articles and review papers to identify any additional studies that could contribute to the overall understanding of nosocomial infections in the Indian healthcare setting [17]. The criteria for inclusion in this review encompassed observational studies, experimental studies, systematic reviews, and meta-analyses that specifically investigated the relationship between nosocomial infections and their implications within the healthcare system of India. It is noteworthy that only studies involving adult human participants were considered, with no specific exclusion criteria outlined [18–24]. The review exclusively focused on peer-reviewed, published articles to maintain a high standard of quality and credibility. Rigorous evaluation of the titles, abstracts, and full-text articles was independently performed by reviewers to determine eligibility, and any discrepancies that arose were meticulously addressed through discussion and consensus among the research team. The primary objective of this extensive literature search was to ensure the incorporation of all pertinent studies and to conduct a comprehensive analysis of the landscape of nosocomial infections in the Indian healthcare context.

1.3 How to Combat Nosocomial Infections

One-third of healthcare-associated infections (HAI) can potentially be averted through the implementation of preventive measures alone; it is crucial to acknowledge that surveillance and prevention constitute the fundamental pillars in the effective management of nosocomial infections within healthcare settings. The process of surveillance encompasses the intricate tasks of data collection, interpretation, and analysis of health-related information, a responsibility typically shouldered by diverse entities such as the Antimicrobial Resistance Surveillance and Research Network of the Indian Council of Medical Research (ICMR) and the National Centre for Disease Control (NCDC). Despite the diligent application of preventive strategies, instances of HAI persist and continue to pose a challenge. The concept of de-escalation, at its core, revolves around the practice of initiating treatment with a broad-spectrum antibiotic, pending the availability of susceptibility test results. This practice is particularly crucial in cases involving critically ill patients, as unwarranted de-escalation could potentially exacerbate the prevailing resistance patterns among bacterial strains [25]. It is imperative to recognize that the prolonged utilization of a specific antibiotic in treating infections within a healthcare setting exerts selective pressure, thereby fostering conditions conducive to the emergence of resistance. On the other hand, the strategy of rotation entails the temporary removal of a specific antibiotic or an entire class of antibiotics from the treatment regimen, aimed at mitigating or stabilizing resistance trends [26–28]. However, within the context of an intensive care unit (ICU) setting, the impact of rotation strategies may not be as profound. Instances of unwarranted de-escalation therapies administered to patients have been correlated with a heightened proliferation of resistant bacterial strains. Failure to promptly adapt treatment regimens to address this evolving scenario may lead to a further deterioration of the situation. It is a widely acknowledged fact that prevention is unequivocally superior to cure, underscoring the critical importance of curtailing the incidence of HAI. Thus, a comprehensive assessment of the prevailing trends in HAI prevalence across various tertiary care facilities in India, alongside an evaluation of existing management protocols, is imperative to fully grasp the gravity and implications associated with HAI occurrences.

The management of the spread of healthcare-associated infections (HAI) is contingent upon our comprehensive understanding of the causative organism and the meticulous planning of strategies aimed at containment. In the United Kingdom, the national surveillance service oversees a prominent initiative that consolidates the data pertaining to reported HAIs into a unified database, facilitating the continuous monitoring of our progress in HAI control and the predominant organisms implicated during a specific timeframe. The findings of a survey conducted in 2002 highlighted intravenous catheters as the primary source of bacteremia, underscoring their significance in the transmission of infections. Approximately 40% of HAIs can be mitigated through stringent sanitation practices involving the proper handling of contaminated equipment, such as adhering to protocols for protection against bodily fluids, utilizing gloves, masks, and aprons, particularly among healthcare personnel, employing catheter tunneling techniques and favoring the subclavian vein over the internal jugular and femoral veins. The administration of appropriate antibiotic therapy plays a crucial role in combating HAIs, with targeted antibiotics being particularly effective once the susceptibility profile of the causative agent is determined, thereby reducing the risk of antibiotic resistance development. Additionally, the isolation of infected patients, guided by judicious clinical decision-making, contributes significantly to the containment efforts. Furthermore, the implementation of routine surveillance measures in intensive care units (ICUs) by seasoned microbiologists has the potential to yield a reduction in the overall disease burden, thus emphasizing the importance of continuous monitoring and strategic interventions in the ongoing battle against HAIs.

1.4 Susceptible Patients to HAI

This concept pertains to inherent characteristics that inherently drive the patient toward the development of the disease in question. It prompts us to pivot toward a proactive approach in situations where the patient's immune system is compromised or when there is a heightened susceptibility to the ailment. The tools at our disposal for evaluating the severity of the preexisting condition include the Acute Physiology and Chronic Health Evaluation (APACHE) score and the diagnosis-related groups, both of which serve as valuable metrics in determining the extent of the illness at hand. The presence of the treating hospital and the personnel involved in the management of patients could potentially contribute as an additional factor to the risk of healthcare-associated infections (HAI). The utilization of various medical devices during the course of treatment serves as a conduit for the transmission of these pathogenic microorganisms either from the external environment or from one anatomical site to another within the body. Consequently, the duration of medical interventions involving these devices is meticulously determined based on the specific clinical requirements and in alignment with the overarching policies formulated at both the institutional and central levels. Surgical Site Infections (SSI) represent a significant burden in the realm of HAI control and necessitate heightened vigilance and adherence to stringent protocols. Additionally, various environmental factors are known to exert a subtle yet noteworthy influence on the overall dynamics of HAI transmission and prevention strategies.

1.5 Causative Organisms

A cluster of pathogenic microorganisms, specifically Enterococcus faecium, Staphylococcus aureus, *Klebsiella pneumoniae*, *Acinetobacter baumannii*, *Pseudomonas aeruginosa*, and *Enterobacter* species, collectively known as ESKAPE pathogens, are responsible for the majority of healthcare-associated infections (HAI) according to a study [20]. When considering the prevalence of HAI, it is observed that *Escherichia coli* and *Staphylococcus aureus* are the most commonly found pathogens; however, their predominant sites of infection exhibit notable differences as highlighted in a previous publication [10]. Recent findings indicate a rising trend in antimicrobial resistance among gram-negative bacteria such as *Klebsiella*, *Pseudomonas*, and *Enterobacter*. This escalation in resistance patterns has raised concerns due to the vast array of antimicrobial agents available for treatment. Noteworthy is the case of *Klebsiella*, where resistance is attributed to the significant variability observed in the plasmid-mediated sulfhydryl reagent variable (SHV1) gene, thereby contributing to the development of resistance mechanisms. Similarly, within the *Enterobacter* species, there has been a gradual emergence of chromosomal type 1 beta-lactamase, resulting in resistance to a broad spectrum of antimicrobials including imipenem. It is worth mentioning that isolates obtained from intensive care units (ICUs) are more frequently targeted for surveillance compared to those from non-ICU settings. The substantial financial investments required for conducting research studies and developing novel pharmaceutical agents by industry stakeholders play a pivotal role in driving up healthcare costs within the system. Consequently, the introduction of newer therapeutic agents tends to be accompanied by higher price tags in comparison to older medications, thereby limiting their accessibility to a broader patient population. Merely focusing on developing new drugs in response to the emergence of resistance among existing agents may not offer a sustainable solution, as it is imperative to ensure a diverse range of antibiotic options remains available for clinical use [10].

1.6 Surveillance

According to the Centers for Disease Control and Prevention (CDC), there exist different types of healthcare-associated infections (HAI). Among these, medical device-associated HAIs stand out as the most prevalent, with approximately 90% of cases being of bacterial origin. The distribution of these infections among individual bacterial species exhibits a certain degree of variability and evolution over time. For instance, the relative incidence rates attributed to *Streptococcus*, coagulase-negative *Staphylococcus*, and coagulase-positive *Staphylococcus* have shown fluctuations, with these pathogens regaining prominence in the landscape of HAIs. Conversely, the occurrences of infections caused by *Klebsiella pneumoniae* and *Escherichia coli* witnessed a decline between the decades spanning from the 1960s to the 1980s. A research endeavor originating from Japan shed light on the specific microbial contributions to primary infections, unveiling that gram-negative anaerobic bacteria bear the greatest burden. *Enterococcus* emerged as the second most common culprit, trailing behind *Streptococcus* and *Staphylococcus* within the realm of gram-positive aerobes. On the other hand, among the gram-negative aerobes, *Escherichia coli*, *Klebsiella*, *Pseudomonas*, and *Enterobacter* were identified as significant contributors to the overall prevalence of HAIs.

Staphylococcus aureus, commonly known as *S. aureus*, is a bacterium that is typically found colonizing approximately 20% of individuals in a normal state.

However, individuals with compromised immune systems are particularly vulnerable to infections caused by *S. aureus*. The infections associated with this bacterium can affect various layers of tissues, ranging from superficial to deep tissues. Furthermore, diseases caused by toxins produced by *S. aureus* include food poisoning and toxic shock syndrome, attributed to enterotoxin and toxic shock syndrome toxin 1 (TSST-1). The mode of transmission for *S. aureus* infections primarily occurs through skin contact and contaminated objects known as fomites.

Escherichia coli, also referred to as *E. coli*, is a type of gram-negative bacteria that is commonly implicated in the development of urinary tract infections (UTIs), septicemia, pneumonia, and meningitis. These infections are largely mediated by the presence of endotoxins, type 3 secretion systems, and the bacterial capsule. The transfer of *E. coli* infections typically transpires from person to person through various mediums such as the environment, food, and water sources.

Vancomycin-resistant enterococci (VRE) are a subset of bacteria that are part of the normal flora in the female genitourinary system. However, in patients undergoing surgical procedures, these bacteria can lead to infections by utilizing their hemolysin and surface protein gelatinase.

Klebsiella, another type of bacteria, is known to colonize the gastrointestinal tract (GIT) and can result in severe conditions such as septicemia and pneumonia. The pathogenic effects of *Klebsiella* are primarily attributed to endotoxins, cell wall components, and polysaccharides. Infection with *Klebsiella* commonly occurs through the contamination of hospital equipment and via person-to-person transmission.

Pseudomonas is a bacterium that is notorious for causing healthcare-associated infections (HAI) with significant mortality rates, particularly affecting the renal, urinary, and respiratory systems. Incubators and sink areas have been identified as common sources of contamination by *Pseudomonas*.

Clostridium difficile, a bacterium that is a typical colonizer, is also a major cause of HAI, particularly responsible for colitis. Remarkably, the spores of *Clostridium difficile* exhibit resistance to standard disinfection practices. The transmission of this bacterium is often facilitated by healthcare personnel. Notably, there has been a noticeable rise in the contribution of *Clostridium difficile* to the incidence of HAI. Surveillance activities play a crucial role in monitoring and interpreting nosocomial data to guide healthcare practices effectively. By analyzing trends and data, healthcare facilities can implement necessary measures to uphold the quality of healthcare delivery. The involvement of microbiology laboratories is pivotal in enhancing the surveillance of HAI by ensuring the accuracy and reliability of results through the implementation of strategies outlined by infection control programs. Establishing high-performance laboratory standards, engaging trained personnel in surveillance programs, and maintaining rigorous monitoring of lab outcomes while utilizing resources judiciously are of paramount importance. Some of the hospital-acquired infections along with the causative organisms are depicted in Table 1.1.

Table 1.1 Showing causative organism of HAI

Hospital-acquired infection	Causative organism
Surgical site infections	*Staphylococcus aureus*, *Pseudomonas* sp., *Escherichia coli*, *Staphylococcus faecalis*, enterococcus, coagulase-negative *Staphylococcus*, *Enterobacter* species
Septicemia	*Staphylococcus aureus*, *Escherichia coli*, *Klebsiella* sp. *Streptococcus pneumoniae*
Gastrointestinal infection	*E. coli*, *Aeromonas* spp. *Plesiomonas shigelloides*, *Clostridium difficile*
Pneumonia	*P. aeruginosa*, *Staphylococcus aureus*, methicillin-susceptible *S. aureus* (MSSA), and methicillin-resistant *S. aureus* (MRSA)
Urinary tract infection	*Enterobacteriaceae*, *Klebsiella*, streptococci, *Enterococci*, *Escherichia coli*

1.7 Epidemiology

The comprehensive examination of the prevalence of healthcare-associated infections (HAI) necessitates meticulous data gathering from the specific cohort of patients whose length of stay in the intensive care unit (ICU) surpasses 48 h. This process involves not only the collection of data but also the meticulous categorization of patients based on various parameters such as the site of infection, the type of infection, the specific microorganism responsible for the infection along with its susceptibility to antibiotics, the age group of the patient, the distinction between nosocomial and non-nosocomial infections through a combination of microbiological and clinical assessments, the calculation of the Acute Physiology and Chronic Health Evaluation (APACHE) score, as well as the conduction of environmental sampling from different surfaces like floors, walls, and other areas potentially contaminated with the patient's fomites. Furthermore, it necessitates the documentation of all medical interventions employed in the management of the affected patient including procedures like catheterization and intubation. Lastly, a thorough analysis of the collected data is performed in comparison to a control group of patients who have not been affected by HAIs [29–31].

A detailed retrospective examination was carried out on the medical reports from the intensive care unit (ICU) at Smt. Kashibai Navale Medical College and General Hospital located in Pune, India, spanning a duration of 1 year as obtained from the literature review of articles. It was found that among the 537 records reviewed, a total of 366 case reports with a duration of stay exceeding 48 h were scrutinized. Within this subset, it was identified that 9.6% of the patients (32 individuals with 35 infections) had developed nosocomial infections, with respiratory tract infections (RTI) emerging as the most prevalent, closely followed by urinary tract infections (UTI). Notably, *Acinetobacter* was identified as the primary causative organism in RTIs, with 21% of the cases exhibiting multidrug resistance. *Pseudomonas*, the second most common pathogen responsible for RTIs and a significant contributor to UTIs, displayed a resistance prevalence of 7.1%. Treatment predominantly involved the administration of penicillins, with patients affected by HAIs experiencing an average ICU stay of 16.5 days, a stark contrast to the shorter duration of 6.4 days observed in unaffected individuals. The respective mortality rates stood at 28.1% for HAI patients and 31.2% for non-affected individuals [29].

1.8 Strategies

The declaration of antimicrobial resistance as a threat to global health security in 2014 by the World Health Organization (WHO) marked a significant milestone in public health discourse. There is a recognized need for enhancement in the availability of data concerning healthcare-associated infections (HAI). Noteworthy is the recent unveiling of a comprehensive 5-year action plan on antimicrobial resistance, a pivotal initiative under the Ministry of Health and Family Welfare (MoHFW) of the Government of India. This plan, known as the Antimicrobial Resistance Surveillance and Research Network, was established in 2013 and 2014 by the Indian Council of Medical Research (ICMR) and the National Centre for Disease Control (NCDC), respectively. Central to this network is the coordination of 25 laboratories scattered across the nation, mandated to consistently furnish reports on the susceptibility and resistance profiles of various highly resistant pathogens. The meticulous oversight conducted by proficient experts, including those at esteemed medical institutions like the Jai Prakash Narayan Apex Trauma Center of All India Institute of Medical Sciences (AIIMS), ensures the meticulous development and implementation of protocols, utilizing data emanating from top-tier laboratories. This meticulous process results in the production of high-caliber data pertinent to healthcare-associated infections (HAI).

The surveillance efforts also extend to the monitoring of medical device interventions, underscored by a long-term goal of bolstering institutional capabilities in infection control through robust task force training initiatives and the amplification of existing programs. This strategic approach ultimately fortifies our ability to effectively counteract outbreaks of healthcare-associated infections (HAI). Nonetheless, the current scope of these endeavors remains somewhat constrained, prompting the imperative for a swift and extensive expansion that encompasses all private and public healthcare facilities.

The accreditation and endorsement bestowed by the National Accreditation Board for Hospitals and Healthcare Providers (NABH) and the National Health Mission (NHM) serve to augment the surveillance capabilities concerning healthcare-associated infections (HAI) within the country. In essence, the overarching objective of these meticulously devised programs is to fortify the landscape of patient safety, firmly establishing it as the foremost priority and ultimate goal [32].

Nanotechnology has recently emerged as a promising approach for drug delivery and enhancement of therapeutic outcomes, with notable progress seen in the incorporation of nanoparticles, particularly those of metallic nature, attributed to their exceptional stability. The utilization of these nanoparticles aims to enhance the permeability of bacterial membranes, consequently leading to an increased uptake of antibiotics by bacterial cells. This mechanism further involves the modification of bacterial signal transduction pathways, induction of free radical damage, as well as the inhibition of oxidative phosphorylation processes. Moreover, the field of nanomedicine, a burgeoning sector within nanotechnology, strives to provide highly specific treatments targeting particular sites, facilitate the delivery of drugs with poor absorption and solubility profiles, and enable sustained drug release to impede biofilm formation [33].

1.9 Conclusion

Hospital-acquired infections (HAIs) significantly impact the mortality rates of patients within intensive care unit (ICU) settings, thereby contributing to an unnecessary healthcare burden. Consequently, it becomes imperative to thoroughly consider all relevant aspects and factors that could mitigate the incidence of such infections across healthcare facilities. The formulation and implementation of robust infection control initiatives at various levels including national, state, and institutional levels, necessitate a synchronized approach. The integration of a microbiology laboratory into the comprehensive management and surveillance protocols can offer valuable insights for epidemiological investigations concerning infection prevalence at the hospital level. Furthermore, the judicious prescription of antibiotics post-sensitivity analysis, whenever feasible, holds promise in bolstering HAI management efforts and curbing the emergence of drug-resistant strains. In essence, prioritizing prevention as the fundamental strategy across all scenarios and environments is paramount in effectively managing HAIs.

References

1. Chahardehi AM, Ghasemi AH. Improving management of hospital-acquired infections in the healthcare setting using antimicrobial coating. Life Sci. 2023;1:23–39.
2. Singh S, Shahadah A, Kumari G, Priya P. Hospital acquired infections during patient incubation at tertiary care hospital of northern India. Int J Med Sci Clin Res Stud. 2023;3:407–12.
3. Goyal M, Chaudhry D. Impact of educational and training programs on knowledge of healthcare students regarding nosocomial infections, standard precautions and hand hygiene: a study at tertiary care hospital. Indian J Crit Care Med. 2019;23:227–31.
4. Mythri H, Kashinath K. Nosocomial infections in patients admitted in intensive care unit of a tertiary health center, India. Ann Med Health Sci Res. 2014;4:738–41.
5. Inweregbu K, Dave J, Pittard A. Nosocomial infections. BJA Educ. 2005;5:14–7.
6. Saba N, Balwan W. Study of frequency, epidemiology of nosocomial infections in healthcare centres. Saudi J Pathol Microbiol. 2023;8:160–6.
7. Girou E, Stephan F, Novara A, Safar M, Fagon JY. Risk factors and outcome of nosocomial infections: results of a matched case-control study of ICU patients. Am J Respir Crit Care Med. 1998;157:1151–8.

8. Robinson ML, Johnson J, Naik S, et al. Maternal colonization versus nosocomial transmission as the source of drug-resistant bloodstream infection in an Indian neonatal intensive care unit: a prospective cohort study. Clin Infect Dis. 2023;77:S38–45.
9. Sahu MK, Siddharth B, Choudhury A, et al. Incidence, microbiological profile of nosocomial infections, and their antibiotic resistance patterns in a high volume cardiac surgical intensive care unit. Ann Card Anaesth. 2016;19:281–7.
10. Emori TG, Gaynes RP. An overview of nosocomial infections, including the role of the microbiology laboratory. Clin Microbiol Rev. 1993;6:428–42.
11. Khan HA, Ahmad A, Mehboob R. Nosocomial infections and their control strategies. Asian Pac J Trop Biomed. 2015;5:509–14. https://www.sciencedirect.com/science/article/pii/S2221169115000829.
12. Akhtar N. Hospital acquired infections in a medical intensive care unit. J Coll Physicians Surg Pak. 2010;20:386–90. https://web.archive.org/web/20170811182357id_/https://www.jcpsp.pk/archive/2010/Jun2010/9.pdf.
13. Swaminathan S, Prasad J, Dhariwal AC, et al. Strengthening infection prevention and control and systematic surveillance of healthcare associated infections in India. BMJ. 2017;358:j3768.
14. Murhekar MV, Kumar CG. Health-care-associated infection surveillance in India. Lancet Glob Health. 2022;10:e1222–3.
15. Mathur P, Malpiedi P, Walia K, et al. Health-care-associated bloodstream and urinary tract infections in a network of hospitals in India: a multicentre, hospital-based, prospective surveillance study. Lancet Glob Health. 2022;10:e1317–25.
16. Chacko B, Thomas K, David T, Paul H, Jeyaseelan L, Peter JV. Attributable cost of a nosocomial infection in the intensive care unit: a prospective cohort study. World J Crit Care Med. 2017;6:79–84.
17. Mateescu MC, Grigorescu S, Socea B, Bloanca V, Grigorescu OD. Contribution to the personalized management of the nosocomial infections: a new paradigm regarding the influence of the community microbial environment on the incidence of the healthcare-associated infections (HAI) in emergency hospital surgical departments. J Pers Med. 2023;13:210.
18. Raoofi S, Pashazadeh Kan F, Rafiei S, et al. Global prevalence of nosocomial infection: a systematic review and meta-analysis. PLoS One. 2023;18:e0274248.
19. Chandra P, Anburaj SE, Vijayanarayana K, et al. Outcome and attributable cost associated with bacterial resistant infections in a tertiary care hospital. J Appl Pharm Sci. 2023;13:132–40.
20. Chakraborty M, Sardar S, De R, et al. Current trends in antimicrobial resistance patterns in bacterial pathogens among adult and pediatric patients in the intensive care unit in a tertiary care hospital in Kolkata, India. Antibiotics (Basel). 2023;12:459.
21. Rosenthal VD, Myatra SN, Divatia JV, et al. The impact of COVID-19 on health care-associated infections in intensive care units in low- and middle-income countries: International Nosocomial Infection Control Consortium (INICC) findings. Int J Infect Dis. 2022;118:83–8.
22. Biondo C, Ponzo E, Midiri A, Ostone GB, Mancuso G. The dark side of nosocomial infections in critically ill COVID-19 patients. Life (Basel). 2023;13:1408.
23. Ramasamy C, Narayan G, Mishra AK, John KJ, Lal A. Nosocomial infections in COVID-19 patients treated with immunomodulators: a narrative review. Front Biosci (Schol Ed). 2022;14:26.
24. Samia NI, Robicsek A, Heesterbeek H, Peterson LR. Methicillin-resistant staphylococcus aureus nosocomial infection has a distinct epidemiological position and acts as a marker for overall hospital-acquired infection trends. Sci Rep. 2022;12:17007.
25. Ananda T, Modi A, Chakraborty I, Managuli V, Mukhopadhyay C, Mazumder N. Nosocomial infections and role of nanotechnology. Bioengineering (Basel). 2022;9:51.
26. Neog N, Phukan U, Puzari M, Sharma M, Chetia P. Klebsiella oxytoca and emerging nosocomial infections. Curr Microbiol. 2021;78:1115–23.
27. Sharma A, Thakur A, Thakur N, Kumar V, Chauhan A, Bhardwaj N. Changing trend in the antibiotic resistance pattern of Klebsiella pneumonia isolated from endotracheal aspirate samples of ICU patients of a tertiary care hospital in north India. Cureus. 2023;15:e36317.

28. Sinha S, Behera S. Time to place Clostridium difficile infections in major healthcare-associated infections list. Indian J Crit Care Med. 2023;27:152–3.
29. Pradhan NP, Bhat SM, Ghadage DP. Nosocomial infections in the medical ICU: a retrospective study highlighting their prevalence, microbiological profile and impact on ICU stay and mortality. J Assoc Physicians India. 2014;62:18–21. https://pubmed.ncbi.nlm.nih.gov/25906516/.
30. Choudhuri AH, Chakravarty M, Uppal R. Epidemiology and characteristics of nosocomial infections in critically ill patients in a tertiary care intensive care unit of northern India. Saudi J Anaesth. 2017;11:402–7.
31. Shalini S, Kranthi K, Gopalkrishna BK. The microbiological profile of nosocomial infections in the intensive care unit. J Clin Diagn Res. 2010;4:3109–12. https://www.jcdr.net/articles/PDF/932/1032_1211_E(C)_F(J)_R(J)_PF_p.pdf.
32. Edwardson S, Cairns C. Nosocomial infections in the ICU. Anaesth Intensive Care Med. 2018;20:14–8.
33. Kumar A, Rai A. Prevalence of surgical site infection in general surgery in a tertiary care centre in India. Int J Surg. 2017;4:3101–6.

Chapter 2
Prevalence, Etiology, and Disease Burden

2.1 Introduction

In order to provide prevalence and incidence rate estimates that are deemed to be both reliable and generalizable, it is imperative for studies to encompass a sample size that is sufficiently large to capture the majority, if not all, of the cases. Furthermore, this sample must be adequately distributed, both in terms of geographical locations and sociological factors, so as to be truly representative of the general population being studied. When dealing with rare diseases, such as many autoimmune rheumatic diseases, the challenge is significantly amplified due to the scarcity of cases and the inherent difficulty in locating them. Consequently, these unique circumstances dictate the necessity for surveys that cover even larger populations in order to obtain stable estimates, as well as requiring longer periods of observation to accurately gauge incidence rates. Naturally, the expansion in population coverage leads to a proportional increase in the financial costs, time commitment, and overall effort that are essential for the execution of such comprehensive studies. Given the complexities involved, it is not surprising that studies relying on primary data collection methods to ascertain the prevalence and incidence of diseases like systemic lupus erythematosus (SLE) are relatively uncommon in the scientific literature.

Understandably, researchers and investigators have been diligently exploring alternative approaches to circumvent the aforementioned challenges while still ensuring the validity and reliability of their estimates. Among the various strategies considered, one particularly promising avenue involves the utilization of administrative data that incorporate diagnosis codes. Administrative data sets are essentially collections of data that are gathered for purposes such as monitoring, reimbursement, or regulatory compliance, typically overseen by governmental bodies or insurance providers, and not primarily intended for research endeavors. Nevertheless, the sheer breadth and depth of information contained within administrative databases often encompass substantial proportions of the population under study.

R. Chakraverty, A. K. Kundu, *Hospital-Acquired Infections in Intensive Care Unit and their Management*, https://doi.org/10.1007/978-981-96-0018-2_2

Studies of disease prevalence and incidence involve three main activities that are crucial in the research process: the initial step of assembling the cohort to be studied, followed by the meticulous task of sorting individuals into affected and unaffected groups through a process known as case ascertainment, and, finally, accurately counting the number of individuals affected by the disease under investigation. The predominant focus of methodological research in the utilization of administrative data for the purpose of estimating disease prevalence and incidence has been directed toward assessing the validity of case ascertainment within these particular data sources [1]. Various factors such as coding errors, instances of "rule-out" diagnoses, and constraints associated with the number of diagnoses that are included in a given dataset can potentially introduce inaccuracies into administrative data, leading to variations in accuracy levels across different data sources. While the act of counting individuals affected by a disease may appear to be a straightforward process, innovative capture-recapture methods have been developed to examine the possibility of a significant undercount and to provide estimates for the number of missing cases [2]. Surprisingly, there has been relatively limited attention given to exploring how the process of assembling the cohort might influence the calculated rates of disease prevalence and incidence.

It is essential to recognize that the settings exposing individuals to potential HCAIs include a wide range of environments such as acute care hospitals, home care services, ambulatory care centers, nursing homes, and family medicine clinics. These infections are known to manifest within a specific timeframe ranging from 48 h up to as long as 30 days subsequent to a patient's initial admission to a healthcare facility. It is crucial to note that the environments predisposing individuals to potential exposure to HCAIs encompass a diverse range of settings including, but not limited to, acute care hospitals, home care services, ambulatory care centers, nursing homes, as well as family medicine clinics. The various forms of healthcare-associated infections encompass a spectrum of conditions such as central line-associated bloodstream infections, which occur when a catheter is inserted directly into a vein leading to the heart, catheter-associated urinary tract infections characterized by infections affecting the urinary system in relation to the presence of a catheter, surgical site infections that typically arise at the location where a surgical intervention was conducted, and ventilator-associated pneumonia which denotes a lung infection that develops in patients who are undergoing respiratory ventilator support [3].

2.2 Prevalence

The prevalence of hospital-acquired infections (HCAIs) in India, as reported by the International Nosocomial Infection Control Consortium, stands at approximately 9.06 infections per 1000 intensive care unit (ICU) patient days. This rate of infection can exhibit significant variations, ranging from 4.4% to 83.09% across different hospitals in India, surpassing the rates observed in comparably affluent nations as highlighted by Iyer, Sewlikar, and Desai in 2015. The elevated prevalence of HCAIs in India not only leads to increased morbidity and mortality rates among patients but also imposes a substantial economic burden on the healthcare system of the country, as noted. Patients afflicted with HCAIs often encounter exorbitant financial implications due to prolonged hospitalization periods necessitated by their conditions [4].

A comprehensive investigation tracking HCAIs within a tertiary care public hospital disclosed that the average duration of hospital stay for HCAI patients, after being matched with controls based on age and gender, exceeded that of non-HCAI patients by 11.96 days, as elucidated by Babbar, Biswal, Digamber, and Gupta in 2019. Consequently, the cumulative expenses incurred by both the patient and the healthcare facility may surge to two to four times the costs associated with treating a non-infected patient, as highlighted by Satpathy, Chaudhry, Gupta, and Kapil in 2013 [5]. A patient diagnosed with an HCAI who necessitates intensive care unit confinement in a hospital could potentially face a daily financial outlay reaching up to INR 223,155.81 (equivalent to approximately USD 2932.81), as stated by Kumar, Jithesh, and Gupta in 2016.

Moreover, individuals grappling with HCAIs may confront escalated risks of enduring long-term disabilities and developing resistance to antimicrobials and antibiotics in the aftermath of their illnesses. The multifaceted health and financial challenges posed by HCAIs are not easily alleviated in the short run, as emphasized by Babbar and colleagues in 2019. In essence, the detrimental impact of HCAIs on the Indian healthcare system manifests through amplified healthcare expenditures, compromised care quality, and adverse effects on patient health outcomes, thus underscoring the profound harm inflicted by these infections [6].

2.3 Enhancing the Efficiency of Sanitation Methods [7]

The primary reason behind the transmission of healthcare-associated infections (HCAIs) to patients within hospitals in India can be attributed to inadequate sanitation procedures being followed. Hospital personnel who mistakenly perceive direct contact with patients during routine medical examinations, such as taking blood pressure readings, conducting temperature screenings, or touching an item within a patient's room as still being sterile, may unintentionally elevate the likelihood of HCAIs due to the transfer of bacteria from one patient to another [5]. The implementation of effective sanitation measures stands as a crucial element in the prevention of HCAIs, with numerous research studies highlighting a notable decrease in HCAI transmission between patients when healthcare workers adhere to proper hand hygiene protocols like handwashing or utilizing alcohol-based disinfectants before and after interacting with patients [8].

Regrettably, there exists a substantial knowledge disparity between theoretical understanding and practical application in numerous hospital settings. All individuals, ranging from janitorial staff to practicing physicians, possess a comprehension of what constitutes appropriate sanitary practices, yet a considerable portion express doubts regarding their efficacy. This skepticism is often coupled with a deficiency in accessible resources. For example, in a qualitative analysis carried out at a rural teaching hospital, many healthcare professionals voiced a preference for conventional soap over alcohol-based sanitizers. Moreover, washbasins and hand sanitizers are not readily obtainable, with staff members highlighting the impracticality of sterilizing equipment and their hands when moving between patients on a regular basis. The optimal scenario of a hospital staff member being able to wash their hands 20–30 times daily is hindered by factors, such as inadequate clean water supply, overcrowded hospital premises, and inadequate staffing levels [9].

Regarding handwashing methodologies, research indicates that practices can vary significantly among hospital staff due to a multitude of factors, including individual experience, personal beliefs, societal norms, and peer influence. This discrepancy is further exacerbated by a lack of rigorous administrative supervision, resulting in the proliferation of misinformation and a diversion of focus. The institution of compulsory educational seminars for hospital employees to familiarize them with optimal handwashing protocols and strategies for minimizing infection transmission can substantially contribute to mitigating the risk of HCAIs at the grassroots level [10].

2.4 Accountability Frameworks

The importance of accountability in the realm of healthcare-associated infections (HCAIs) risk reduction practices is just as significant as the emphasis placed on education within this context. Implementation of a robust infrastructure that enables healthcare staff to consistently report data regarding the incidence of HCAIs among patients not only fosters a sense of accountability but also serves to reinforce the established guidelines. Numerous institutions have documented the existence of HCAIs; however, the enforcement of a zero-tolerance policy (with the overarching objective being the complete eradication of patient cases of HCAIs) remains somewhat lacking. The procedures for reporting accountability facilitate the engagement of various stakeholder groups (such as administrators, policymakers, healthcare professionals, and patients) in discussions aimed at instigating transformative actions to achieve the ultimate goal of zero instances of HCAIs among patients [6].

The issue of accurately reporting HCAIs and instigating change is also influenced by the fear of reprisal. Hospital personnel may harbor concerns about facing punitive measures if the incidence of HCAIs escalates within a healthcare facility, which could lead them to deliberately refrain from diagnosing patients with HCAIs (opting instead for less severe diagnoses) or neglect to escalate HCAI cases to higher authorities. Consequently, critical information relating to the state of a hospital's environmental hygiene standards may be lost. Conversely, hospital administrators may encounter obstacles in the form of local media channels. The apprehension of media coverage triggering community backlash has contributed to instances of falsified HCAI data being reported. Nevertheless, media exposure may also act as a catalyst for enhancing public awareness about HCAIs, compelling hospitals to assume accountability for proactively addressing the risks posed by HCAIs to residents in their localities [11].

To tackle these challenges effectively, the implementation of a robust "national benchmarking system for HCAIs with transparent public disclosure of outcomes" is imperative. Presently, there exists a significant disparity in hospital accreditation, with numerous healthcare facilities failing to adhere to the established guidelines of health agencies such as the Indian Public Health Standards, Indian Council of Medical Research protocols, and Kayakalp guidelines. These guidelines comprehensively outline protocols for managing HCAIs; however, there is currently no regulatory framework in place mandating hospitals to adhere to and report on infection control outcomes. Furthermore, previous legislations like the Clinical Establishments (Registration and Regulation) Act, 2010, have only been adopted at the state level and lack mandatory enforcement at the national level [5].

Therefore, the national government's increasing emphasis on the necessity for hospitals to uphold accreditation licenses that are under strict regulation by the established National Accreditation Board for Hospitals and Healthcare Providers (NABH) is paramount in ensuring quality healthcare provision. It is noteworthy that at present, a mere 714 hospitals hold accreditation from the NABH, a figure that represents a significantly small proportion when juxtaposed with the extensive number of hospitals across India. The proposal to introduce internal infection control committees within each hospital setting emerges as a strategic approach toward fostering standardized monitoring of healthcare-associated infections (HCAIs) that can be tailored to meet the specific requirements of individual hospitals while concurrently aligning with a comprehensive national surveillance initiative linked to accreditation protocol (Centers for Disease Control and Prevention, 2021). Nevertheless, there exists a pressing need for a concerted regional endeavor to engage with public hospitals situated in rural regions catering to underserved communities. It is insufficient to solely impose a nationwide directive, assuming that small-scale hospitals with limited financial resources can effortlessly adhere to impeccable infection control benchmarks. The practical challenges encountered at the grassroots level, including overcrowding in rural healthcare facilities, understaffing issues, and deficiencies in access to basic amenities such as clean water and soap, demand a multifaceted approach encompassing targeted funding initiatives and educational campaigns designed not only for healthcare personnel but also for members of the community.

The current cultural framework pertaining to health practices holds significant potential in serving as a robust foundation for the advancement of sanitation measures and the reduction of healthcare-associated infections (HCAIs) at a community level. One noteworthy cultural tradition in India, which has often been overlooked by mainstream modern medical institutions, is Ayurveda—an ancient holistic system of medicine that places emphasis on bodily imbalances and stress as key factors contributing to the onset of diseases and ailments (Johns Hopkins Medicine). This 3000-year-old system commands an equal level of reverence from many Indians as Western medicine, with ongoing research efforts focusing on various Ayurvedic products like herbs, minerals, and metals. Despite the intricate nature of Ayurveda that remains not entirely comprehended, numerous studies have highlighted the significance and efficacy of traditional Ayurvedic botanical products in cleansing and sterilizing environments. A study conducted in 2019 showcased the efficacy of garlic peel, turmeric powder, ajwain seed powder, and loban fumigation in disinfecting surfaces contaminated with drug-resistant methicillin-resistant *Staphylococcus aureus* (MRSA) bacteria, a strain commonly associated with nosocomial (hospital-acquired) infections. Given the challenge posed by the limited accessibility and affordability of conventional disinfecting products, a potential solution lies in further exploring the properties of Ayurvedic preparations to equip rural healthcare facilities with widely recognized, efficient natural Ayurvedic remedies that are readily available in most villages. Moreover, rural communities may exhibit a greater receptivity toward traditional, familiar disinfection practices coupled with proper sanitation protocols, rather than the introduction of Western sanitizing agents. By addressing this cultural disparity, enhanced adherence to sanitation measures within local communities can be facilitated [12].

2.5 Conclusion

In conclusion, it is imperative that a dual approach to instigating change is adopted simultaneously at both the national and local levels in order to effectively address healthcare-associated infections (HCAIs) at the individual level. The implementation of highly stringent government-mandated structural directives would establish a benchmark for medical sanitation protocols; nevertheless, one must also acknowledge the impracticality of anticipating a comprehensive dissemination of changes without the integration of behavioral modification strategies. At the local level, there exists a pressing need for a concerted and unwavering effort toward educational outreach initiatives tailored to cater to the specific requirements of the community, rather than adhering to a generic, one-size-fits-all model. Particularly in rural settings, there is a critical necessity to place greater emphasis on the incorporation of traditional Ayurvedic methodologies alongside conventional Western medical practices. The recognition of the enduring significance of non-Western biomedical wisdom in addressing global health challenges serves to dismantle apprehensions surrounding contemporary medical procedures and facilitates the alignment of disparate sanitation frameworks sharing common foundational principles. Amidst the backdrop of strained healthcare infrastructures burdened with limited resource capacities, the implementation of such behavioral interventions holds promise for widespread adoption, extending beyond the confines of India. In essence, by embracing these methodologies, healthcare systems can transcend the conventional ethos of merely abiding by the principle of "do no harm" and, instead, strive toward eradicating the adverse impact of HCAIs while enhancing the overall well-being of patients.

References

1. Furst DE, Clarke AE, Fernandes AW, Bancroft T, Greth W, Iorga SR. Incidence and prevalence of adult systemic lupus erythematosus in a large U.S. managed-care population. Lupus. 2013;22:99–105.
2. Widdifield J, LaBrecque J, Lix L, et al. A systematic review and critical appraisal of validation studies to identify rheumatic diseases in health administrative databases. Arthritis Care Res. 2013;65:1490. https://doi.org/10.1002/acr.21993.
3. Anand C. When hospitals infect you. The Hindu; 2017.
4. Allegranzi B, Pittet D. Role of hand hygiene in healthcare-associated infection prevention. J Hosp Infect. 2009;73(4):305–15.
5. Satpathy S, Chaudhry A, Gupta SK, Kapil A. P261: study of hospital associated infections (HAI) at tertiary hospital in India; economic implication for developing countries. Antimicrob Resist Infect Control. 2013;2:1.
6. Balusu C. Addressing the prevalence of healthcare-associated infections in India. Undergrad J Public Health. 2022;6.
7. Babbar P, Biswal M, Digamber B, Gupta A. Healthcare associated infections in intensive care units: a pilot study in a tertiary care public hospital in India. J Prev Infect Control. 2019;5(1):1.
8. Bhatwalkar SB, Shukla P, Srivastava RK, Mondal R, Anupam R. Validation of environmental disinfection efficiency of traditional Ayurvedic fumigation practices. J Ayurveda Integr Med. 2019;10(3):203–6.
9. Biswal M, Mewara A, Appannanavar SB, Taneja N. Mandatory public reporting of healthcare-associated infections in developed countries: how can developing countries follow? J Hosp Infect. 2015;90(1):12–4.
10. Centers for Disease Control and Prevention. Types of healthcare-associated infections. Centers for Disease Control and Prevention; 26 March 2014. http://www.cdc.gov/hai/infectiontypes.html.
11. Diwan V, Gustafsson C, Rosales Klintz S, Joshi SC, Joshi R, Sharma M, Shah H, Pathak A, Tamhankar AJ, Stålsby LC. Understanding healthcare workers self-reported practices, knowledge and attitude about hand hygiene in a medical setting in rural India. PLoS One. 2016;11(10):e0163347.
12. Swaminathan S, Prasad J, Dhariwal AC, Guleria R, Misra MC, Malhotra R, Mathur P, Walia K, Gupta S, Sharma A, Ohri V. Strengthening infection prevention and control and systematic surveillance of healthcare associated infections in India. BMJ. 2017;58:358.

Chapter 3
Current Management Algorithms of Hospital-Acquired Infections

3.1 Introduction

Healthcare-associated infections (HAIs) refer to infections contracted by patients while receiving medical or surgical care. These occurrences are a frequent complication in healthcare settings, often stemming from multidrug-resistant microorganisms due to excessive antibiotic use. HAIs are associated with heightened morbidity and mortality rates, prolonged hospitalizations, and increased healthcare expenditures. The monitoring of endemic HAIs is essential for comprehending their consequences, pinpointing vulnerable demographics and procedures, and directing interventions to diminish their occurrence. The surveillance of HAIs is a critical component of global infection prevention and control initiatives. Nonetheless, the efficacy of HAI surveillance hinges on the adoption of standardized definitions. The definitions utilized in surveillance systems such as the National Healthcare Safety Network (NHSN) or the European Centre for Disease Prevention and Control (ECDC) are complex, necessitating specific resources and expertise in diagnostics, epidemiology, and infection control. Consequently, in 2010, only 16% of low-income and middle-income countries (LMICs) had established comprehensive HAI surveillance at either national or subnational levels [1].

The chapter delves into the significance of establishing a national-level surveillance system for healthcare-associated infections (HAI), such as ventilator-associated pneumonia and surgical site infection. The authors underscore the necessity to broaden and sustain the surveillance system instigated by Mathur and colleagues in order to facilitate prompt identification and containment of outbreaks resulting from emerging infectious diseases and multidrug-resistant organisms. The document also underscores the importance of validating the adjusted case definitions utilized in the research prior to their widespread implementation. Furthermore, the authors accentuate that the surveillance system will furnish valuable data on antimicrobial resistance, which can guide local, regional, and national antimicrobial

R. Chakraverty, A. K. Kundu, *Hospital-Acquired Infections in Intensive Care Unit and their Management*, https://doi.org/10.1007/978-981-96-0018-2_3

resistance stewardship strategies and endeavors. Additionally, the document proposes that integrating this surveillance system with global platforms, such as the Global Antimicrobial Resistance and Use Surveillance System, will promote the exchange of knowledge and dissemination of optimal practices for infection prevention and control. In essence, the article highlights the imperative to institute and enhance a national-level surveillance system for significant healthcare-associated infections. This system is envisioned to not only offer crucial data on antimicrobial resistance but also to facilitate the prompt identification and containment of outbreaks induced by both established and emerging infectious diseases and multidrug-resistant organisms. The emphasis lies on the significance of validating the adjusted case definitions used in the research before their broader implementation. Furthermore, the document underscores the potential advantages of connecting the surveillance system with global platforms in terms of disseminating best practices for infection prevention and control [2].

3.2 Importance of Quality Indicators in Healthcare Assessment

The evaluation of the efficiency of healthcare through diverse quality markers such as the successful treatment of illnesses, enhancement of longevity, and enhancement of overall well-being is a crucial element. This underscores the significance of upholding a collection of benchmarks and recommendations in the management of patients and the effective allocation of healthcare assets to assess the standard of healthcare. Furthermore, it underscores that the quality can also be assessed through the examination of patient results and technical proficiency. It is imperative to consider these factors when gauging the overall effectiveness and quality of healthcare services provided to individuals.

3.3 Involvement of Organizations in Defining and Measuring Quality [3–8]

Moreover, the active participation of numerous entities in establishing and evaluating the standards of excellence in the healthcare sector, along with overseeing its implementation, holds significant importance. This includes entities like the Joint Commission in the United States, the Care Quality Commission in the United Kingdom, and the National Accreditation Board for Hospitals and Healthcare Providers (NABH) in India, which are responsible for granting accreditation to healthcare facilities that demonstrate a commitment to providing high-quality healthcare services. These organizations serve as key players in ensuring that healthcare providers adhere to stringent quality standards and continuously strive to improve the delivery of healthcare services to meet the evolving needs of patients and society.

3.4 Significance of Quality Indicators in Healthcare Evaluation

Overall, this underscores the significance of quality indicators in assessing the effectiveness of healthcare, the role of established standards and guidelines, and the involvement of organizations in ensuring and accrediting the delivery of quality healthcare services. It provides an overview of the various aspects and considerations in evaluating and monitoring the quality of healthcare, laying the groundwork for further exploration and understanding of this critical area in the field of healthcare delivery.

3.5 Healthcare-Associated Infections (HAI) Risks and Costs [9–12]

The article explores the risk dimensions of healthcare-associated infections (HAI) and the significant costs associated with these infections to the health service. It emphasizes that the impacts of HAI are not limited to financial costs and patient stays but are multidimensional. The financial costs incurred by patients with HAI are substantially higher, with patients staying in hospitals for two to five times longer than uninfected patients, resulting in an average of 11 additional days per case.

3.6 Nonfinancial Implications of HAI

The article underscores that the consequences of HAI extend beyond financial implications to encompass nonfinancial penalties that can have both immediate and long-term effects. These nonfinancial penalties are often overlooked but are equally important. Although they are challenging to measure, their recognition is crucial. The complexity and stability of the present situation underline the necessity for a sustained, focused, and professional risk management approach to improve the HAI situation. The article thus highlights the need to consider both the obvious and less obvious costs and implications of HAI, emphasizing the importance of a multidimensional perspective for a comprehensive understanding of the impacts of these infections [13].

3.7 Comprehensive Understanding and Holistic Approach to HAI

This provides a comprehensive overview of the substantial costs and multidimensional impacts of HAI on the health service. It emphasizes the need for a holistic approach to HAI that considers not only the financial costs and immediate consequences but also the nonfinancial penalties that can have enduring effects on patients and the healthcare system as a whole. The article underscores the significance of recognizing and addressing the less obvious costs associated with HAI and advocates for a sustained and professional risk management approach to effect tangible improvements in this critical area. The article delves into the topic of hospital-acquired infections (HAIs) or healthcare-associated infections, which refer to infections that are contracted during a hospitalization period and were not present at the time of admission. HAIs encompass a variety of infections such as catheter-associated urinary tract infections, central line-associated bloodstream infections, surgical site infections, ventilator-associated pneumonia, hospital-acquired pneumonia, and *Clostridium difficile* infections. The document elucidates the signs and symptoms that may suggest the presence of an HAI, which can include symptoms like productive cough, shortness of breath, abdominal pain, altered mental status, and various other indicators. The identification and understanding of these symptoms are crucial for timely diagnosis and appropriate management of HAIs to improve patient outcomes and prevent further complications in healthcare settings [14].

3.8 Objectives

The main goals of this chapter are to provide a detailed explanation of the pathophysiology of healthcare-associated infections (HAIs), examine the various laboratory tests that are employed in assessing these infections, present an overview of their management strategies, and emphasize the significance of enhancing care coordination within the interprofessional team to effectively curtail the spread of infections and improve the delivery of care for patients affected by HAIs. The paper emphasizes the need for a multidisciplinary approach involving various healthcare professionals to address HAIs effectively. Pathophysiology of HAIs: This discusses the various mechanisms through which HAIs can occur, such as direct contact, ingestion, inhalation, and transmission by fomites. It explores the role of microbial factors, host factors, and environmental factors in the development of these infections. Additionally, it highlights the importance of infection control measures and surveillance in preventing and controlling the spread of HAIs within healthcare settings [15].

3.9 Laboratory Tests for Evaluation

The discussion on laboratory tests for evaluation provides a comprehensive overview of the various laboratory tests employed in assessing hospital-acquired infections (HAIs). These tests play a crucial role in the diagnosis and management of HAIs by providing valuable information on the causative pathogens and their susceptibility patterns. Understanding the results of these tests is essential in guiding healthcare professionals in prescribing appropriate antimicrobial therapy and implementing infection control measures to prevent the spread of HAIs within healthcare settings, including blood cultures, urine cultures, wound swabs, and molecular diagnostic tests. It emphasizes the significance of accurate and timely diagnostic testing in identifying the causative pathogens and guiding appropriate treatment strategies for HAIs [16].

3.10 Management of HAIs

In the realm of managing HAIs, a multifaceted approach is essential, which includes adherence to the principles of antimicrobial stewardship, implementation of robust infection control practices, and tailoring antibiotic therapy based on the susceptibility profiles of the identified pathogens. Moreover, the significance of adopting preventive strategies like promoting hand hygiene, ensuring proper environmental sanitation, and judicious use of medical devices cannot be overstated in mitigating the risk of HAI transmission and improving patient outcomes [17].

3.11 Improving Care Coordination

Improving Care Coordination: This underscores the need for effective collaboration among the interprofessional team, including physicians, nurses, infection control practitioners, and other healthcare providers, to improve care coordination and prevent the transmission of HAIs. It emphasizes the role of education, communication, and the establishment of standardized protocols in enhancing the overall management of patients affected by HAIs. It provides a comprehensive overview of the pathophysiology, evaluation, management, and care coordination related to HAIs. It emphasizes the importance of a coordinated and interdisciplinary approach to effectively address these infections and improve patient outcomes within healthcare settings [18].

3.12 Hospital-Acquired Infections (HAIs)

The research paper delves into the intricate domain of hospital-acquired infections (HAIs), colloquially known as healthcare-associated infections, which are contracted post-hospitalization and typically become evident 48 h after admission. Noteworthy is the vigilant surveillance conducted by entities such as the National Healthcare Safety Network (NHSN) to thwart HAIs and enhance patient welfare. The paper delineates various categories of HAIs, encompassing central line-associated bloodstream infections (CLABSI), catheter-associated urinary tract infections (CAUTI), surgical site infections (SSI), hospital-acquired pneumonia (HAP), ventilator-associated pneumonia (VAP), and *Clostridium difficile* infections (CDI), elucidating their clinical implications and management strategies [19–22].

Furthermore, the discourse underscores the escalating emphasis placed by healthcare facilities on infection monitoring systems and prevention tactics to curb the incidence of HAIs. The repercussions of HAIs reverberate not only at the individual patient level but also permeate to the community sphere, given their association with multidrug-resistant pathogens. Identifying individuals with predisposing factors for HAIs and multidrug-resistant organisms assumes paramount importance in preempting these infections and curtailing their dissemination, underscoring the critical role of proactive surveillance and intervention in safeguarding public health [23–25].

The chapter delves into the modifications in the criteria for characterizing pneumonia, emphasizing the identification of patients vulnerable to multidrug-resistant pathogens to prevent the excessive use of antibiotics. It highlights the transition from the previously employed term healthcare-acquired pneumonia (HCAP) to hospital-acquired pneumonia (HAP) as stipulated by the Infectious Disease Society of America (IDSA). Moreover, ventilator-associated pneumonia (VAP) is described as pneumonia that emerges more than 48–72 h after endotracheal intubation. Both HAP and VAP are linked with unfavorable outcomes, substantial morbidity, and mortality on a global scale. In essence, the chapter provides a thorough examination of hospital-acquired infections, their supervision and monitoring, the significance of preventive measures, and the revised criteria for recognizing and handling pneumonia, specifically HAP and VAP, to enhance patient outcomes and curtail the dissemination of multidrug-resistant infections.

3.13 Risk Factors Contributing to Hospital-Acquired Infections [26]

The susceptibility to hospital-acquired infections (HAIs) is impacted by various elements such as infection control practices at the establishment, the immune status of the patient, and the prevalence of pathogens in the community. Individuals with compromised immune systems, advanced age, extended hospitalizations, multiple underlying health conditions, frequent visits to healthcare facilities, mechanical ventilation, invasive procedures, and tenure in an intensive care unit (ICU) face heightened risks of contracting HAIs. Furthermore, the administration of intravenous antibiotics within the preceding 90 days stands out as a significant risk factor for the development of resistance to multiple antimicrobial agents. A prevalence study demonstrated that roughly 19.5% of ICU patients had at least one HAI, signifying an elevated risk for individuals in these wards. Common microorganisms responsible for HAIs encompass *Clostridium difficile*, *Candida* spp., *Enterobacteriaceae*, staph aureus, *Enterococcus*, *Pseudomonas*, proteus, *Klebsiella*, and *E. coli*. These pathogens can induce particular forms of HAIs like *Clostridium difficile* colitis (CDI), central line-associated bloodstream infections (CLABSI), catheter-associated urinary tract infections (CAUTI), surgical site infections (SSI), hospital-acquired pneumonia (HAP), and ventilator-associated pneumonia (VAP). Grasping the prevalent pathogens linked with distinct types of HAIs is imperative for the efficacious implementation of preventive and control measures within healthcare settings.

3.14 Strategies to Combat Hospital-Acquired Infections

Furthermore, hospitalizations play a crucial role in the management of acute illnesses; however, they also heighten the vulnerability of patients to acquiring nosocomial infections, which are often antimicrobial-resistant, from various sources within the healthcare setting such as other patients, hospital staff, or the facility itself. It is imperative to emphasize the prevention and control of healthcare-associated infections (HAIs) like *Clostridium difficile* infection (CDI), central line-associated bloodstream infection (CLABSI), catheter-associated urinary tract infection (CAUTI), surgical site infection (SSI), hospital-acquired pneumonia (HAP), and ventilator-associated pneumonia (VAP) as a means to alleviate the impact of these infections on both patients and healthcare systems. Effective strategies to combat HAIs encompass strict adherence to infection control protocols, prudent utilization of antimicrobial agents, and continuous surveillance of these infections to track patterns and detect emerging threats. Understanding the specific pathogens associated with each type of HAI is important for tailoring prevention and control measures to target the most significant sources of transmission, thereby reducing the incidence of these infections in healthcare settings. The findings underscore the importance of comprehensive infection control practices and vigilance in identifying and addressing risk factors for HAIs to safeguard patients and healthcare workers from the adverse effects of these infections.

3.15 Recommendations for Preventing Hospital-Acquired Infections

In conclusion, the risk for HAIs in healthcare facilities is influenced by a combination of factors such as infection control practices, patient immune status, and pathogen prevalence in the community. Specific patient populations, such as those in the ICU, are at a higher risk for HAIs. Furthermore, the surveillance and comprehension of the predominant pathogens linked to specific types of HAIs are fundamental in devising successful prevention and control interventions. The research outcomes underscore the significance of robust infection control practices and targeted measures to reduce the risk of HAIs and safeguard the well-being of patients and healthcare personnel from the adverse effects of such infections. A comprehensive study conducted by the Centers for Disease Control and Prevention (CDC) involved a multistate point prevalence analysis of healthcare-associated infections (HAIs) in 2014, encompassing 11,282 patients across 183 hospitals in the United States. The results of the investigation unveiled that around 4% of hospitalized patients contracted at least one HAI. Statistical data from 2011 indicated that an estimated 648,000 patients admitted to hospitals encountered a total of 721,800 infections. The most prevalent types of infections, listed in descending order, included pneumonia, surgical site infections, gastrointestinal infections, urinary tract infections (UTIs), and primary bloodstream infections, with catheter-associated bloodstream infections being a significant subset.

3.16 Leading Pathogens and Prevention Efforts

The predominant pathogens responsible for causing HAIs were identified as *Clostridium difficile*, *Staphylococcus aureus*, *Klebsiella*, and *Escherichia coli*. Notably, *Staphylococcus aureus*, including the methicillin-resistant *Staphylococcus aureus* (MRSA) strain, was predominantly associated with skin and surgical site infections. The seminal SENIC study shed light on the potential to reduce infections by a substantial margin, up to one-third, through the amalgamation of infection surveillance and control initiatives. The report recognized a certain decline in the occurrence of specific HAIs attributable to heightened awareness and the implementation of robust preventive measures within hospital environments. The diligent surveillance of infections and the implementation of preventive strategies have yielded positive outcomes in the prevention of HAIs, as evidenced by a notable 46% decrease in the rates of central line-associated bloodstream infections (CLABSI) between the years 2008 and 2013.

3.17 Impact and Importance of Infection Surveillance

The findings underscore the significant burden of HAIs on hospitalized patients and the healthcare system, with a considerable number of patients affected by these infections annually. The specific identification of dominant pathogens causing HAIs provides valuable insights for targeted preventive and control measures. Additionally, the potential for a substantial reduction in infections through comprehensive infection tracking and control programs highlights the importance of proactive measures in healthcare settings. The positive impact of infection surveillance and prevention practices in reducing the incidence of certain HAIs emphasizes the potential for further advances in this area.

In conclusion, the study sheds light on the prevalence of HAIs and their associated pathogens in the US healthcare system. It underscores the need for continued efforts to implement and strengthen infection surveillance and prevention practices to mitigate the burden of HAIs on patients and reduce the associated healthcare costs. While progress has been made in reducing certain HAIs, ongoing research and implementation of effective strategies are crucial for further advancements in this critical area of healthcare.

The topic delves into the intricacies of pathogen transmission within healthcare environments, shedding light on the various risk factors linked to specific instances of hospital-acquired infections (HAIs). Among these risk factors, *Clostridioides difficile* infection (CDI) is influenced by recent antibiotic usage, gastric acid suppressants, nonsteroidal anti-inflammatory drugs, and certain comorbidities. Conversely, surgical site infections (SSI) are impacted by patient-related elements like age, diabetes, obesity, as well as operative factors such as procedure duration and antimicrobial prophylaxis. Catheter-associated urinary tract infections (CAUTI) can arise through intraluminal colonization, periurethral spread, and biofilm formation. Similarly, central line-associated bloodstream infections (CLABSI) entail colonization, biofilm formation, and migration mechanisms. The prevalence of multidrug-resistant (MDR) pathogens stands out as a significant contributor to HAIs, resulting in prolonged hospitalization, heightened mortality rates, and increased healthcare expenses. Notably, MDR pathogens are notably linked to healthcare-associated pneumonia (HAP) and ventilator-associated pneumonia (VAP), with septic shock, extended hospital stays, and recent intravenous antibiotic administration emerging as pivotal risk factors for MDR VAP. These findings underscore the intricate nature of diverse risk factors associated with various HAIs, underscoring the critical importance of targeted prevention and control strategies to mitigate their impact on healthcare facilities.

3.18 Impact of Acute Illness on Drug Pharmacokinetics and Pharmacodynamics

The article discusses the impact of acute illness, particularly sepsis, on the toxicokinetics, pharmacokinetics, and pharmacodynamics of drugs, with a focus on the dosing of renal-excreted medications and antibiotics. During an acute illness, the volume of distribution of a drug can vary, affecting dosing considerations. This significance is particularly pronounced in the context of medications like aminoglycosides and beta-lactams. The estimation of glomerular filtration rate (eGFR), which might be compromised during sepsis, is also underscored as a vital determinant in establishing appropriate medication dosages for critically ill patients. Noteworthy guidelines from the Infectious Diseases Society of America (IDSA) and the American Thoracic Society (ATS) advocate for the selection of antibiotic dosages based on pharmacokinetic and pharmacodynamic principles for critically ill patients grappling with ventilator-associated pneumonia.

Additionally, the article emphasizes that the effectiveness of antibiotics can be contingent on factors such as concentration (e.g., fluoroquinolones and aminoglycosides), time (e.g., beta-lactams), or a combination of both (e.g., vancomycin). To uphold therapeutic concentrations, time-dependent medications are typically administered as prolonged infusions, while concentration-dependent drugs are prescribed aiming for a single high peak (via a high one-time dose) or multiple peaks with intermittent dosing.

3.19 Considerations for Antibiotic Dosing in Hospital-Acquired Infection

Regarding hospital-acquired infection (HAI), the article's focus on the impact of acute illness and sepsis on drug dosing is crucial. In the context of HAI, critically ill patients are often vulnerable to infections, and the appropriate dosing of antibiotics is essential for effectively treating these infections. The article emphasizes the need to consider the altered toxicokinetic and pharmacokinetics during acute illness when determining medication dosing for patients with HAI. By understanding the changes in drug distribution and renal function during sepsis, healthcare providers can optimize antibiotic dosing to effectively combat HAI in critically ill patients.

Overall, this article underscores the importance of considering the specific pharmacokinetic and pharmacodynamic changes that occur during acute illness, particularly in the context of HAI. By tailoring drug dosing to account for these changes, healthcare providers can optimize the treatment of HAI in critically ill patients, ultimately contributing to better patient outcomes and reduced rates of HAI.

3.20 Importance of Detailed Patient History and Physical Examination

The topic underscores the significance of acquiring a detailed patient history and conducting a thorough physical examination to differentiate between infections acquired prior to admission and those acquired in the hospital setting. It emphasizes that symptoms like subjective fever, chills, and night sweats may suggest a non-hospital-acquired infection, while common infectious symptoms encompass fever, chills, altered mental status, productive cough, and various localized pains. Vital signs such as hypothermia or hyperthermia, tachypnea, tachycardia, and hypotension could indicate a systemic inflammatory response or sepsis. The assessment of external devices like catheters, endotracheal tubes, and intravascular lines is vital, along with details regarding their location and insertion.

3.21 Scrutiny of Medical Devices and Surveillance for Infections

The chapter underscores the importance of reassessment and potential replacement of hastily inserted central lines within 24–48 h, particularly if inserted under aseptic conditions or in the presence of new fever during hospitalization, as central venous catheters serve as a significant origin of hospital-acquired bloodstream infections. Furthermore, catheter-associated urinary tract infections and ventilator-associated pneumonia are recognized as other origins of bloodstream infections. The daily inspection of surgical sites and breaches in skin integrity is advised to promptly detect evolving infections, manage them effectively, and reduce complications. Additionally, a thorough examination of the abdomen and stool samples is often required in the assessment for *Clostridium difficile* infection. The scholarly document provides an in-depth analysis of the importance of detailed patient history, comprehensive physical examination, and scrutiny of medical devices in the identification and management of hospital-acquired infections.

3.22 Article Emphasizes the Importance of Laboratory Testing

The aforementioned scholarly article accentuates the significance of laboratory testing in aiding the identification of potential infection sources and evidence of organ dysfunction. It suggests that serum levels of lactic acid, liver transaminases, prothrombin time, BUN, and serum creatinine can corroborate clinical observations of hypoperfusion. Moreover, the article underscores other critical laboratory findings such as white cell counts, bands, thrombocytopenia, hypoglycemia, hyperglycemia, and reduced mixed venous blood saturation.

3.23 Significance of Obtaining Samples for Cultures

The importance of procuring specimens for microbial cultures prior to the commencement of antibiotic therapy is emphasized in the article, highlighting its crucial role in promptly identifying the causative microorganism and determining its susceptibility to antimicrobial agents. Such data is instrumental in guiding the transition from the use of broad-spectrum antibiotics to more targeted therapeutic options tailored to combat the specific pathogens encountered, ultimately leading to enhanced clinical outcomes for patients. By facilitating the selection of appropriate antimicrobial treatments based on the pathogen's susceptibility profile, this practice aids in optimizing patient care and mitigating the risks associated with indiscriminate antibiotic use.

3.24 Recommendations Against Unnecessary Investigations

Moreover, the article cautions against conducting investigations that do not influence clinical decision-making or the clinical trajectory. It emphasizes that in cases where the pretest probability of hospital-acquired infection (HAI) such as ventilator-associated pneumonia (VAP) is high, ancillary tests like C-reactive protein (CRP) and procalcitonin are considered supplementary and not recommended.

3.25 Noninvasive Sampling in Hospital-Acquired Pneumonia

Regarding patients with hospital-acquired pneumonia (HAP) or VAP, the article highlights that recent guidelines advocate for noninvasive sampling through tracheal aspirates. Research has demonstrated that this method yields results of comparable quality to invasive techniques like quantitative tracheal lavage or bronchoscopy.

To summarize, the article underscores the significance of laboratory testing in enhancing the history and clinical examination for pinpointing the infection source and organ dysfunction. It underscores the necessity of obtaining cultures prior to commencing antibiotic treatment to facilitate prompt detection of pathogens and their susceptibility to antimicrobials. Furthermore, the article offers insights into ancillary test usage and advocates for noninvasive sampling approaches for specific hospital-acquired infections, ultimately contributing to the enhancement of patient care and treatment optimization within the realm of hospital-acquired infection.

3.26 Management of Hospital-Acquired Infections and Sepsis

The management of hospital-acquired infections, especially within the realm of sepsis, comprises a variety of essential elements that are crucial for successful outcomes. Within standard goal-directed therapy, there are multiple key actions involved, including the administration of antibiotics, fluid resuscitation, and diligent monitoring to detect any signs of organ dysfunction. Following the implementation of fluid resuscitation, it becomes of utmost importance to consistently perform serial evaluations to assess both the clinical and hemodynamic responses exhibited by the patient. The criticality of selecting the appropriate antibiotics and determining the optimal timing for their initiation cannot be overstated in the effective management of these types of infections. The decision-making process surrounding the choice and timing of antibiotic administration plays a pivotal role in ensuring positive patient outcomes. In the context of empiric antibiotics, it is crucial to base the selection on the individual patient's specific risk factors for multidrug-resistant

(MDR) pathogens, as well as their overall clinical condition and stability. There is a strong emphasis on the necessity of promptly initiating antibiotic therapy, with the recommended timeframe being ideally within an hour of suspicion of infection. In situations where there is a suspicion of a central line-associated bloodstream infection, it is advised to procure two separate sets of blood cultures, with one obtained from a peripheral venous site and the other from the central venous catheter site, before commencing antibiotic treatment. Additionally, in instances of hypotension, hypoperfusion, or organ dysfunction, it is absolutely imperative to swiftly remove the catheter and promptly send the tip for culture analysis to facilitate appropriate management strategies.

3.27 Protocol for Catheter-Associated Infections and Preventative Strategies

In situations where there is suspicion of catheter-associated urinary tract infections (CAUTIs), it is imperative to adhere to specific protocols as per established guidelines and recommendations. The initial step involves the removal of the existing catheter, followed by the collection of a urine sample from the newly inserted catheter, ideally prior to the commencement of antibiotic therapy, in order to optimize the likelihood of obtaining valuable microbiological data. These meticulous steps have been demonstrated to significantly improve the yield of microbiological specimens, thereby aiding in accurate diagnosis and subsequent treatment. Furthermore, in alignment with universal precautions for infection control, it is crucial that all types of catheters, be they central lines or urinary catheters, are promptly removed when they are no longer deemed necessary for the patient's care. With regard to the management of catheter-associated UTIs, the generally recommended duration for administering antibiotics is around 7 days, although in instances where there is a delayed clinical response or presence of bacteremia, an extension of the antibiotic course to 10–14 days may be warranted. Strategies aimed at preventing CAUTIs encompass a variety of interventions such as reducing the frequency of catheter usage, minimizing the duration of catheter dwelling, employing antimicrobial-coated catheters, and judiciously implementing antibiotic prophylaxis in specific clinical scenarios. In a broader context, the effective control and management of nosocomial infections demand a comprehensive and multifaceted approach that involves timely and judicious use of antibiotics, appropriate catheter care practices, and strict adherence to infection prevention strategies.

The discourse further delves into the optimal duration of antibiotic therapy regimens for hospital-acquired pneumonia (HAP) and ventilator-associated pneumonia (VAP), emphasizing that a standard 7-day course is typically sufficient unless there are compelling clinical reasons necessitating a longer treatment duration. It is essential that these antibiotic regimens possess efficacy against common pathogens implicated in pneumonia, including *Staphylococcus aureus* and *Pseudomonas aeruginosa*, to ensure successful resolution of the infection. Additionally, the article underscores the importance of tailoring antibiotic selection when dealing with multidrug-resistant (MDR) pathogens, advocating for the use of alternative agents that demonstrate activity against these resilient organisms, as opposed to relying solely on traditional antibiotics with limited effectiveness against such strains.

3.28 Preventive Strategies for CLABSI

The article delves into the topic of central line-associated bloodstream infections (CLABSI) and discusses the decline in their incidence in the United States, attributing this trend to the adoption of evidence-based preventive measures. These interventions encompass a range of strategies, including the meticulous observance of aseptic protocols during catheter insertion, the timely removal of unnecessary catheters, the use of chlorhexidine baths, the application of antimicrobial dressings, and the administration of catheter lock solutions. Moreover, it underscores the significance of tailoring the duration of antibiotic therapy for CLABSI based on factors such as the complexity of the infection, the status of the catheter (retained or removed), and whether complications are present.

3.29 Treatment Options for *Clostridium difficile* Infection

In addition, the article sheds light on *Clostridium difficile* infections, highlighting oral vancomycin as the preferred treatment option and recommending adjustments to the initial antibiotic regimen in cases of primary infection. It also presents metronidazole as a viable alternative medication, while newer options like fidaxomicin are also brought into focus. Furthermore, the article acknowledges ongoing investigations into the efficacy of other antibiotics such as teicoplanin. Notably, fecal microbiota transplantation is mentioned as a last-resort intervention for severe and resistant cases of *Clostridium difficile* infection. Specifically, the article offers valuable insights into the optimal antibiotic regimens for hospital-acquired pneumonia (HAP) and ventilator-associated pneumonia (VAP), outlines preventive strategies and antibiotic duration considerations for CLABSI, and discusses the various therapeutic approaches available for managing *Clostridium difficile* infections. These comprehensive findings play a crucial role in guiding clinical decision-making processes and enhancing patient outcomes in the management of these infectious diseases.

3.30 Importance of Antibiotic Prophylaxis and Skin Decontamination

The article emphasizes the critical importance of proper hand hygiene and infection prevention strategies when caring for surgical sites postoperatively. It stresses the significance of antibiotic prophylaxis and skin decontamination in preventing surgical site infections (SSI). Specifically, it highlights the necessity of employing antibiotics to cover common pathogens early, with subsequent adjustments based on culture reports. The recommendation to initiate antibiotics for coverage against *Staphylococcus aureus* and other pathogens, including *Pseudomonas*, is a crucial aspect based on the clinical situation. It is also important to highlight the significance of considering antibiotics that have efficacy against multidrug-resistant (MDR) organisms, such as MRSA and carbapenemase-producing *Enterobacteria*, in specific instances.

3.31 Universal Standard Infection Control Measures

Furthermore, the emphasis is placed on the necessity of universal standard infection control practices in addition to antibiotic prophylaxis and skin decontamination. These practices encompass actions like handwashing using soap and water or utilizing alcohol-based disinfectants before and after every patient interaction. Such measures play a pivotal role in diminishing the rates of transmission of MDR pathogens. The article draws attention to research results that suggest the utilization of gloves and gowns may not always prevent contamination and might not be adequate in halting the spread of infections.

3.32 Comprehensive Overview of Preventing Surgical Site Infections

Overall, the topic provides a comprehensive overview of the essential factors in preventing surgical site infections, including the use of appropriate antibiotics, skin decontamination, and universal standard infection control measures. It emphasizes the need for early and targeted antibiotic prophylaxis, as well as the consideration of MDR pathogens in treatment approaches. Furthermore, it highlights the limitations of certain infection control measures, as evidenced by the findings from the study regarding the use of gloves and gowns.

References

1. Boev C, Kiss E. Hospital-acquired infections: current trends and prevention. Crit Care Nurs Clin North Am. 2017;29(1):51–65.
2. Habboush Y, Yarrarapu SNS, Guzman N. Infection Control. StatPearls [Internet]. Treasure Island: StatPearls Publishing; 2023.
3. Kalil AC, Metersky ML, Klompas M, Muscedere J, Sweeney DA, Palmer LB, Napolitano LM, O'Grady NP, Bartlett JG, Carratalà J, El Solh AA, Ewig S, Fey PD, File TM, Restrepo MI, Roberts JA, Waterer GW, Cruse P, Knight SL, Brozek JL. Management of adults with hospital-acquired and ventilator-associated pneumonia: 2016 Clinical Practice Guidelines by

the Infectious Diseases Society of America and the American Thoracic Society. Clin Infect Dis. 2016;63(5):e61–111.
4. Cillóniz C, Dominedò C, Torres A. An overview of guidelines for the management of hospital-acquired and ventilator-associated pneumonia caused by multidrug-resistant Gram-negative bacteria. Curr Opin Infect Dis. 2019;32(6):656–62.
5. Sydnor ER, Perl TM. Hospital epidemiology and infection control in acute-care settings. Clin Microbiol Rev. 2011;24(1):141–73.
6. Metersky ML, Kalil AC. New guidelines for nosocomial pneumonia. Curr Opin Pulm Med. 2017;23(3):211–7.
7. Stiller A, Schröder C, Gropmann A, Schwab F, Behnke M, Geffers C, Sunder W, Holzhausen J, Gastmeier P. ICU ward design and nosocomial infection rates: a cross-sectional study in Germany. J Hosp Infect. 2017;95(1):71–5.
8. Novosad SA, Fike L, Dudeck MA, Allen-Bridson K, Edwards JR, Edens C, Sinkowitz-Cochran R, Powell K, Kuhar D. Pathogens causing central-line-associated bloodstream infections in acute-care hospitals-United States, 2011–2017. Infect Control Hosp Epidemiol. 2020;41(3):313–9.
9. Flores-Mireles A, Hreha TN, Hunstad DA. Pathophysiology, treatment, and prevention of catheter-associated urinary tract infection. Top Spinal Cord Inj Rehabil. 2019;25(3):228–40.
10. Young PY, Khadaroo RG. Surgical site infections. Surg Clin North Am. 2014;94(6):1245–64.
11. Babcock HM, Zack JE, Garrison T, Trovillion E, Kollef MH, Fraser VJ. Ventilator-associated pneumonia in a multi-hospital system: differences in microbiology by location. Infect Control Hosp Epidemiol. 2003;24(11):853–8.
12. Magill SS, Edwards JR, Bamberg W, Beldavs ZG, Dumyati G, Kainer MA, Lynfield R, Maloney M, McAllister-Hollod L, Nadle J, Ray SM, Thompson DL, Wilson LE, Fridkin SK, Emerging Infections Program Healthcare-Associated Infections and Antimicrobial Use Prevalence Survey Team. Multistate point-prevalence survey of health care-associated infections. N Engl J Med. 2014;370(13):1198–208.
13. Hughes JM. Study on the efficacy of nosocomial infection control (SENIC Project): results and implications for the future. Chemotherapy. 1988;34(6):553–61.
14. Eze P, Balsells E, Kyaw MH, Nair H. Risk factors for *Clostridium difficile* infections—an overview of the evidence base and challenges in data synthesis. J Glob Health. 2017;7(1):010417.
15. Nickel JC, Costerton JW. Bacterial biofilms and catheters: a key to understanding bacterial strategies in catheter-associated urinary tract infection. Can J Infect Dis. 1992;3(5):261–7.
16. del Pozo JL, Patel R. The challenge of treating biofilm-associated bacterial infections. Clin Pharmacol Ther. 2007;82(2):204–9.
17. Bell T, O'Grady NP. Prevention of central line-associated bloodstream infections. Infect Dis Clin N Am. 2017;31(3):551–9.
18. Patel AR, Patel AR, Singh S, Singh S, Khawaja I. Central line catheters and associated complications: a review. Cureus. 2019;11(5):e4717.
19. Serra-Burriel M, Keys M, Campillo-Artero C, Agodi A, Barchitta M, Gikas A, Palos C, López-Casasnovas G. Impact of multi-drug resistant bacteria on economic and clinical outcomes of healthcare-associated infections in adults: systematic review and meta-analysis. PLoS One. 2020;15(1):e0227139.
20. Magiorakos AP, Srinivasan A, Carey RB, Carmeli Y, Falagas ME, Giske CG, Harbarth S, Hindler JF, Kahlmeter G, Olsson-Liljequist B, Paterson DL, Rice LB, Stelling J, Struelens MJ, Vatopoulos A, Weber JT, Monnet DL. Multidrug-resistant, extensively drug-resistant and pandrug-resistant bacteria: an international expert proposal for interim standard definitions for acquired resistance. Clin Microbiol Infect. 2012;18(3):268–81.
21. Kalil AC, Metersky ML, Klompas M, Muscedere J, Sweeney DA, Palmer LB, Napolitano LM, O'Grady NP, Bartlett JG, Carratalà J, El Solh AA, Ewig S, Fey PD, File TM, Restrepo MI, Roberts JA, Waterer GW, Cruse P, Knight SL, Brozek JL. Executive summary: management of adults with hospital-acquired and ventilator-associated pneumonia: 2016 Clinical Practice Guidelines by the Infectious Diseases Society of America and the American Thoracic Society. Clin Infect Dis. 2016;63(5):575–82.

22. Miller SE, Maragakis LL. Central line-associated bloodstream infection prevention. Curr Opin Infect Dis. 2012;25(4):412–22.
23. Mermel LA, Allon M, Bouza E, Craven DE, Flynn P, O'Grady NP, Raad II, Rijnders BJ, Sherertz RJ, Warren DK. Clinical practice guidelines for the diagnosis and management of intravascular catheter-related infection: 2009 Update by the Infectious Diseases Society of America. Clin Infect Dis. 2009;49(1):1–45.
24. Al Momani LA, Abughanimeh O, Boonpheng B, Gabriel JG, Young M. Fidaxomicin vs vancomycin for the treatment of a first episode of Clostridium difficile infection: a meta-analysis and systematic review. Cureus. 2018;10(6):e2778.
25. Furuya EY, Cohen B, Jia H, Larson EL. Long-term impact of universal contact precautions on rates of multidrug-resistant organisms in ICUs: a comparative effectiveness study. Infect Control Hosp Epidemiol. 2018;39(5):534–40.
26. Danna DM. Hospital costs associated with sepsis compared with other medical conditions. Crit Care Nurs Clin North Am. 2018;30(3):389–98.

Chapter 4
Catheter-Associated Bloodstream Infections in the Intensive Care Units

4.1 Introduction

Catheter-related bloodstream infections (CRBSIs) represent a significant challenge within healthcare facilities, accounting for 10–15% of all nosocomial infections, a statistic of considerable importance. Although central vascular catheters are commonly recognized as a primary culprit, the role of peripheral catheters as a source of nosocomial bacteremia [1] is often overlooked, highlighting a gap in existing knowledge. The primary objective of this rigorous analysis is to delve into the epidemiology, clinical implications, and management strategies pertaining to CRBSIs, aiming to provide a comprehensive overview of this critical issue. Notably, the review underscores the substantial attributable mortality rates ranging from 12 to 25% and the prolonged hospitalization periods of 7–15 days linked to these infections, emphasizing the severe impact they have on patient outcomes. Through a meticulous synthesis of current research findings, this review accentuates the pressing necessity for proactive interventions to mitigate the incidence and repercussions of CRBSIs, pointing toward a crucial area for improvement in healthcare systems. Furthermore, the challenges associated with diagnosing and treating CRBSIs are meticulously explored, underscoring the significance of adhering to evidence-based protocols for catheter insertion and maintenance practices, thereby enhancing patient safety. Moreover, the review delves into the pivotal role of antibiotic stewardship programs and infection prevention measures in combating CRBSIs, shedding light on effective strategies for reducing the burden of these infections. Through a comprehensive analysis of the existing literature, the review critically evaluates various interventions designed to alleviate the impact of CRBSIs, offering valuable insights for healthcare practitioners and policymakers alike. In conclusion, the review advocates for a holistic approach encompassing infection control protocols, antimicrobial stewardship initiatives, and enhanced education for healthcare providers to effectively address the challenge posed by CRBSIs. Ultimately, the findings

R. Chakraverty, A. K. Kundu, *Hospital-Acquired Infections in Intensive Care Unit and their Management*, https://doi.org/10.1007/978-981-96-0018-2_4

underscore the urgent need for the implementation of comprehensive strategies aimed at reducing the occurrence of CRBSIs and enhancing patient outcomes in healthcare environments.

4.2 Definition of CLABSI by CDC

Central line-associated bloodstream infections (CLABSI) present a considerable risk to patient safety and are characterized by the isolation of a pathogen from a blood culture in a patient with a central line either at the onset of infection or within 48 h before its manifestation. This study delves into the surveillance criteria for CLABSI as delineated by the Centers for Disease Control and Prevention (CDC) and underscores the significance of precise diagnosis and reporting practices. Moreover, the research delves into the specific parameters used to identify exit site and tunnel infections in the setting of tunneled catheters. It elucidates the attributes of exit site infections, such as localized inflammation and culture-positive exudate, as well as the characteristics of tunnel infections, which encompass inflammation that extends past the exit site, pain, tenderness, and the presence of culture-positive exudate. Comprehending and adhering to these definitions is paramount for efficient surveillance and handling of CLABSI, as it enables the prompt and accurate detection of infections, thereby assisting in the mitigation of further complications and the enhancement of patient outcomes. To conclude, this article underscores the significance of standardized definitions for CLABSI and its related infections, offering valuable insights for healthcare practitioners engaged in the diagnosis and prevention of these critical healthcare-associated infections. In the case of tunneled catheters, the accepted definitions for exit site and tunnel infections are as follows:

4.3 Exit Site Infection and Tunnel Infection

Exit site infections and tunnel infections are common complications associated with catheter use in healthcare settings. Exit site infections are characterized by localized inflammation within 2 cm of the catheter exit site along with culture-positive exudate. On the other hand, tunnel infections involve inflammation extending beyond 2 cm from the exit site, often associated with pain and tenderness along the subcutaneous track and culture-positive exudates that may not be readily visible. This paper comprehensively discusses the clinical manifestations, diagnostic criteria, and management strategies for exit site and tunnel infections. The authors provide a detailed overview of the microbiology and pathogenesis of these infections, emphasizing the importance of early detection and intervention to prevent complications. Additionally, the review highlights various modalities for diagnosis, including the role of microbiological cultures and imaging techniques in differentiating between exit site and tunnel infections. Furthermore, the paper outlines evidence-based treatment approaches, including antimicrobial therapy and catheter removal when necessary, taking into account factors such as the patient's clinical status and predisposing factors. The authors also address the challenges in managing these infections, such as antibiotic resistance and the impact of biofilm formation. Overall, this comprehensive review serves as a valuable resource for healthcare practitioners involved in the care of patients with catheter-related infections, offering evidence-based guidance for the diagnosis and management of exit site and tunnel infections to improve patient outcomes and reduce the burden of catheter-related complications [2].

4.4 Prevalence

Central venous catheter-related bloodstream infections (CRBSI) represent a significant challenge within the healthcare environment, as evidenced by a recent study that highlighted a prevalence rate of 39.25%. Among the causative agents, *Serratia marcescens* emerged as the most frequently isolated organism, accounting for 23.81% of cases, indicating its clinical relevance in CRBSI. The investigation further pointed out that factors such as patients' immunocompromised status and the duration of catheterization played pivotal roles as significant risk factors for the development of CRBSI. Noteworthy, the study identified a concerning methicillin resistance rate of 33.33% among the isolates, highlighting the growing issue of antibiotic resistance in healthcare settings. Moreover, gram-negative bacteria exhibited high levels of resistance to aminoglycosides, fluoroquinolones, and third-generation cephalosporins, posing additional challenges in the management of CRBSI. In comparison to the data from the National Nosocomial Infections Surveillance (NNIS) system by the Centers for Disease Control and Prevention (CDC), the median CRBSI rate in different intensive care units varied from 1.8 to 5.2 per 1000 catheter days, with an overall rate averaging around 25.6%. These findings emphasize the critical importance of implementing robust infection control measures and antimicrobial stewardship programs to combat the increasing burden of CRBSI, particularly in intensive care settings. Central line-associated bloodstream infections (CRSBI) present a significant threat to individuals with underlying health conditions and those undergoing intravascular catheterization procedures. This research delves into potential risk factors associated with CRSBI, including variables such as the technique and location of catheter insertion, the duration and purpose of catheter use, and the administration of parenteral nutrition.

4.5 Risk Factor

Furthermore, local factors like inadequate personal hygiene practices, the use of occlusive transparent dressings, and nasal colonization by *S. aureus* contribute significantly to the risk of CRBSI development. The study also delves into the role of bacterial colonization in the pathogenesis of CRBSI, emphasizing the impact of contiguous infections on CRSBI development. Specific to dialysis patients, the research highlights risk factors such as contamination of dialysate, poor water treatment quality, dialyzer reuse practices, advanced age, higher doses of recombinant human erythropoietin, lower serum albumin levels, peripheral atherosclerosis, and the presence of diabetes mellitus. A comprehensive understanding of these risk factors is imperative for healthcare professionals in the prevention and management of CRSBI.

This in-depth analysis provides valuable insights into the multifaceted nature of CRSBI risk factors, stressing the importance of tailored interventions and preventive strategies. The research outcomes underscore the significance of considering both general and local risk factors, along with patient-specific variables, in the comprehensive approach to preventing and managing CRSBI. Healthcare providers and clinicians must remain vigilant in addressing these risk factors to enhance patient outcomes and reduce the incidence of CRBSI in clinical settings.

4.6 Pathogenesis

Catheter-related bloodstream infections (CRBSI) represent a considerable challenge within healthcare environments, as there are numerous factors that contribute to the development of these infections. In this study, an examination is carried out on the catheter itself and its involvement in four distinct pathogenic processes. These processes include the colonization of the catheter tip and cutaneous tract by skin flora, the contamination of the catheter lumen, the hematogenous seeding of the catheter from another infected site, and the contamination of the lumen with infusate. Furthermore, the research delves into the impact of antibiotic resistance resulting from biofilm formation on the progression of bacteremia. The significance of distinguishing between catheter colonization and true CRBSI is highlighted in the study, emphasizing that a negative sample related to the catheter may be more effective in ruling out CRBSI compared to a positive sample. Specifically, in cases where a blood culture from the catheter yields positive results while the percutaneous blood sample is negative, it is likely indicative of catheter colonization rather than CRBSI. These findings illuminate the complex nature of CRBSI pathogenesis and underscore the critical necessity for precise diagnostic strategies to accurately differentiate between catheter-related colonization and severe bloodstream infections [3].

4.7 Microorganism Associated with Catheter-Related Bloodstream Infections

Organisms linked to CRBSI typically comprise the normal resident flora of the skin at the insertion site, potentially leading to the colonization of the inserted catheter. The colonization of the tip of intravenous catheters is frequently observed in ICU patients and can serve as a perilous source of bacteremia, leading to sepsis and multi-organ failure.

4.7.1 *Bacterial Infections*

Organisms associated with catheter-related bloodstream infections (CRBSI) are typically part of the normal flora present on the skin at the site where the catheter is inserted, potentially resulting in the colonization of the catheter. This colonization of the intravenous catheter tip is a common occurrence in intensive care unit (ICU) patients and can act as a dangerous reservoir of bacteria, ultimately leading to bacteremia, sepsis, and the failure of multiple organs. In this research study, it was found that 64% of the pathogens responsible for CRBSI were gram-positive, while 36% were gram-negative. The most prevalent pathogen causing CRBSI was *Staphylococcus aureus* at 40%, followed by *Pseudomonas aeruginosa* at 16%, coagulase-negative staphylococci at 8%, *Escherichia coli* at 8%, *Klebsiella pneumoniae* at 8%, and *Acinetobacter baumannii* at 4%. Accordingly, gram-positive cocci accounted for 27% of the isolates, while gram-negative bacilli made up 56%. The percentage of gram-negative CRBSI cases was notably higher compared to what is typically reported in hospitals in Western countries a study demonstrated that coagulase-negative staphylococci were present in 50% of CRBSI cases in their study. In an investigation out of a total of 50 CRBSI episodes, 48% were found to be polymicrobial, 32% were attributed to gram-negative bacilli, and 10% were caused by gram-positive organisms. The most frequently isolated organisms were *Klebsiella pneumoniae* at 16%, coagulase-negative staphylococci at 14%, and *Pseudomonas aeruginosa* at 11%.

4.7.2 *Fungal Infection*

Various research investigations have presented varying data on the prevalence of fungal infectious agents that are accountable for catheter-related bloodstream infections (CRBSI), predominantly consisting of yeasts, with no instances of filamentous fungus reported in the literature. For instance, in a study, it was found that 16% of the infectious agents causing CRBSI were identified as *Candida* species. Another study conducted in 2008 also highlighted that the fungal pathogen isolated from central venous catheters (CVC) was predominantly *Candida* at 11.7%. Moreover, a separate study indicated the presence of non-albicans *Candida* species in a single documented case. These findings underscore the significance of understanding the spectrum of fungal pathogens implicated in CRBSI to enhance diagnostic and therapeutic strategies [4].

4.7.3 Viral and Parasitic Infections

The microorganisms causing catheter-related bloodstream infections (CRBSI) typically originate from the skin flora, comprising predominantly of bacteria and yeasts. Conversely, the understanding of the normal viral and parasitic components of skin flora remains limited, with no research demonstrating any viral or parasitic etiology for CRBSI. Detection of CRBSI involves a comprehensive approach encompassing both clinical evaluation and laboratory analysis. The identification of CRBSI is a crucial aspect of patient care, requiring a judicious combination of clinical symptom assessment and laboratory tests to ensure timely and accurate diagnosis.

4.8 Quantitative Paired Blood Culture [5]

Catheter-related bloodstream infection (CRBSI) is characterized by a quantitative blood culture ratio exceeding 5:1 (CVC vs. peripheral) and requires the identification of isolates from positive blood cultures from both peripheral and CVC samples through pulsed-field gel electrophoresis. The diagnosis of CRBSI is established when the colony counts in blood cultures from the CVC are at least three times higher than those from blood drawn from a peripheral vein. The literature presents a range of fold differences between CVC and peripheral blood, typically recommending thresholds between threefold and tenfold. In the presence of an indwelling CVC, the preferred approach for diagnosing CRBSI involves obtaining comparative blood cultures from the CVC and a peripheral vein before starting antibiotic therapy, as suggested by most experts. It is essential to collect cultures from all lumens of the CVC, which is considered the most accurate method for diagnosing CRBSI. When peripheral vein access is not feasible, it is advised to draw two blood samples through different catheter lumens, with a colony count in one sample being at least three times higher than in the other, indicating a potential CRBSI scenario.

4.9 Differential Time to Positivity [6–11]

CRBSI is indicated by the presence of microbial growth in blood samples obtained from a central venous catheter (CVC) at least 2 h prior to the detection of growth in blood samples taken concurrently from a peripheral vein. The majority of modern automated blood culture systems have the capability to promptly furnish this crucial data, thereby indicating a shift toward the incorporation of this test as a routine diagnostic procedure in clinical settings. It is highly probable that the timely identification of CRBSI through this diagnostic approach will soon be established as a standard practice in the field of healthcare.

4.10 Short-Term Catheters, Including Arterial Catheters

For routine clinical microbiological analysis in short-term catheter tip cultures, it is advised to utilize the roll plate technique as recommended in the literature [12]. This method is commonly employed due to its effectiveness in isolating and identifying microbial pathogens present on catheter tips. In cases where there is suspicion of pulmonary artery catheter infection, it is essential to culture the introducer tip to determine the presence of any infectious agents [13]. The culture of the introducer tip is a crucial step in diagnosing and managing infections related to pulmonary artery catheters, allowing for appropriate treatment and prevention strategies to be implemented [14–18].

4.11 Long-Term Catheters

Semiquantitative growth of 15 cfu/catheter segment of the same microbe from both the insertion site culture, and the catheter hub culture strongly indicates a high likelihood that the catheter is the origin of a bloodstream infection. When a venous access subcutaneous port is extracted due to suspected CRBSI, the port is typically transferred to the microbiology laboratory for qualitative culture of the port reservoir contents, along with the catheter tip. This comprehensive approach assists in identifying the specific microorganism responsible for the infection, aiding in targeted treatment strategies and infection control measures. Utilizing these methods can significantly enhance patient care outcomes and minimize the risk of complications associated with catheter-related bloodstream infections [4, 19–22].

4.12 Management of Catheter-Related Bloodstream Infections [23]

The primary goal of conducting regular rounds in the intensive care unit (ICU) by clinical microbiologists and engaging in bedside discussions with intensivists regarding infection management is to ensure timely communication of urgent microbiology results. Such a practice is vital in enabling the initiation of diagnostic, therapeutic, and infection control measures at the earliest opportunity. The comprehensive assessment of infections necessitates a multifaceted approach that encompasses a wide array of historical, epidemiological, clinical, and diagnostic parameters. These parameters include physical examinations, hematological and biochemical investigations, radiological findings, and microbiology results [24].

4.13 Assessment of Infection [25]

Moreover, the clinical microbiology round in the ICU encompasses the interpretation of microbiology findings and providing feedback to the ICU team on antimicrobial resistance patterns. It also involves conducting audits and implementing policies to ensure the rational utilization of diagnostic, therapeutic, and infection prevention/control resources within the unit. In cases of catheter-related bloodstream infections (CRBSI) associated with local or systemic inflammation or immunocompromised states, the prompt removal of catheters is recommended. Antibiotic therapy for catheter-related infections is typically initiated empirically based on factors such as the patient's clinical condition severity, infection risk factors, and probable pathogens linked to the specific intravascular device.

4.14 Infection Prevention and Control [26]

There is a lack of definitive data supporting specific recommendations for the duration of antibiotic therapy for device-related infections. For instance, methicillin-resistant *Staphylococcus aureus* infections may require empirical treatment with vancomycin, while daptomycin could be considered for strains with vancomycin minimum inhibitory concentration values exceeding 2 μg/mL. Empirical coverage for gram-negative bacilli should be tailored according to local antimicrobial susceptibility data and disease severity, potentially involving fourth-generation cephalosporins, carbapenems, or β-lactam/β-lactamase combinations, with or without an aminoglycoside [27].

4.15 General Management

In situations where CRBSI is suspected in critically ill patients with femoral catheters, it is recommended that the initial treatment plan includes a broad spectrum to cover gram-negative bacilli, *Candida* species, and gram-positive pathogens. In the case of suspected catheter-related candidemia, one can consider using *Echinocandins* or fluconazole for empirical treatment [28]. In scenarios where catheter salvage is deemed necessary, it is advisable to opt for antibiotic lock therapy; however, if antibiotic lock therapy is not a feasible option in such circumstances, systemic antibiotics can be administered through a colonized catheter. The likelihood of recurrent bacteremia post-parenteral therapy is higher when the therapy is administered through a catheter that is retained, as opposed to when the catheter is removed, possibly due to suboptimal antibiotic concentrations within biofilms [29]. Strategies aimed at eliminating infections associated with long-term or completely implanted catheters often involve filling the catheter lumen with high concentrations of antibiotics and leaving them in place for extended durations to establish an antibiotic lock. The efficacy of antibiotic lock therapy for CRBSI can vary depending on factors such as the infection site and the causative microorganism. For example, infections in tunnels or pockets may not show a positive response to salvage attempts, whereas coagulase-negative staphylococci are more likely to respond well to antibiotic lock therapy in comparison to *Staphylococcus aureus* [30].

4.16 Antibiotic Lock Therapy and Its Use to Treat Patients with Catheter-Related Infection

Recurrent bacteremia following parenteral treatment presents a higher probability of occurrence when the therapy is administered via a retained catheter as opposed to when the catheter is removed [31]. This phenomenon is believed to be a result of the limited ability of most antibiotics to reach the necessary therapeutic levels required to eliminate microbes that are thriving within a biofilm. In cases where infections are associated with long-term or totally implanted catheters and are predominantly intra-luminal in nature, efforts to eradicate such infections involve filling the catheter lumen with concentrations of antibiotics that exceed therapeutic levels and allowing them to dwell for extended periods, thus establishing an antibiotic lock [32]. The utilization of antibiotic lock therapy for catheter-related bloodstream infections (CRBSI) is typically combined with systemic antibiotic treatment and entails the introduction of a high concentration of an antibiotic, which the causative microorganism is susceptible to, into the catheter lumen. The likelihood of achieving successful outcomes with this approach varies depending on factors such as the location of the infection (e.g., tunnel or pocket infections may not respond well to salvage efforts) and the specific microorganism responsible for the infection (for instance, coagulase-negative staphylococci are more likely to exhibit a positive response, whereas *S. aureus* is usually resistant to such treatment).

4.17 Clinical Presentation

Mild clinical signs of catheter-related bloodstream infection (CRBSI) include feelings of general discomfort and nausea, whereas more severe symptoms are characterized by a high body temperature along with chills, low blood pressure, vomiting, and changes in consciousness. On the other hand, an infection at the exit site of the catheter can be identified by redness, swelling, pain, and the presence of pus draining around the catheter exit, which may extend to a portion of the catheter tunnel external to the cuff. The progression of CRBSI can lead to the development of serious systemic infections and widespread infectious complications, such as infective endocarditis, septic arthritis, osteomyelitis, and abscess formation in the spinal epidural region, which can significantly prolong the duration and severity of the infection. In conclusion, it is important to recognize these different clinical presentations and potential complications associated with CRBSI to facilitate prompt diagnosis and appropriate management strategies in affected individuals.

4.18 Laboratory Diagnosis

Central line-associated bloodstream infections (CLABSIs) are characterized by the presence of at least one positive blood culture from a peripheral vein in a patient with an intravascular catheter, along with clinical signs of infection like fever, chills, or hypotension. The diagnostic criteria for CLABSIs involve various parameters including the isolation of the same organism from both the catheter segment and peripheral blood culture, a positive semiquantitative culture (15 CFU/catheter segment), or a quantitative culture (>10^3 CFU/catheter segment) of the catheter tip. Moreover, a diagnosis of CLABSIs can also be made based on simultaneous quantitative paired blood cultures showing a >5:1 ratio of colony-forming units (CFU) in the central venous catheter (CVC) compared to peripheral blood. In addition to these criteria, a differential time to positivity method may be utilized where a non-quantitative blood culture from the CVC becomes positive at least 2 h earlier than the peripheral blood culture, facilitating the identification of CLABSIs without necessitating catheter removal [33].

In the case of non-tunneled CLABSIs, the catheter responsible for the infection must be promptly removed, even in situations where the definitive diagnostic criteria are not met but clinical suspicion remains high. Conversely, when dealing with long-term catheters, there may be instances where salvage strategies are considered, involving a combination of systemic therapy and an antimicrobial lock (comprising heparin along with a high concentration of an antimicrobial agent selected based on susceptibility testing results). These salvage approaches are typically reserved for specific cases and are aimed at preserving the catheter while effectively treating the infection. These instances include:

Uncomplicated catheter-related bloodstream infections (CLBSI) are typically caused by microorganisms other than *Staphylococcus aureus*, *Pseudomonas aeruginosa*, *Bacillus* spp., fungi, or mycobacteria. This type of infection is commonly observed in patients with limited vascular access sites, especially in those who rely solely on central access for their survival. When dealing with tunneled hemodialysis catheters, uncomplicated exit site infections can often be managed with a brief regimen of either topical or systemic antimicrobials. However, it is crucial to note that all tunnel infections necessitate catheter removal due to the significantly heightened risk of developing CLBSI. Other factors that may indicate the need for CLBSI removal from hemodialysis access sites include the presence of persistent symptoms that endure for more than 36 h, severe sepsis, hemodynamic instability leading to shock, and metastatic infection.

Moreover, cases where blood cultures remain positive even after 72 h of receiving appropriate antimicrobial therapy, or when dealing with challenging-to-treat organisms like *Staphylococcus aureus*, *Pseudomonas*, or fungi, may also require catheter removal. Recurrence of uncomplicated CLBSI, especially in instances where catheters were salvaged due to challenging access issues, could further necessitate removal for effective treatment. In terms of the duration of therapy for patients with uncomplicated CRBSI, in the absence of conditions like endocarditis or metastatic infection, and with negative blood cultures 72 h post-catheter removal, a specific approach to intravenous antimicrobial therapy is recommended based on the causative microorganism.

In cases of *Staphylococcus aureus* infection, a treatment duration of 14 days is advised in the absence of endocarditis. For infections caused by coagulase-negative staphylococci, a shorter therapy course of 7 days is generally sufficient. Enterococci and gram-negative bacilli infections typically require antimicrobial therapy for a duration of 10–14 days. Lastly, infections caused by *Candida* should ideally be treated with a 14-day course of antimicrobials, especially in the absence of retinitis. These specific recommendations aim to guide healthcare providers in optimizing treatment outcomes and minimizing the risks associated with catheter-related bloodstream infections.

4.19 Differential Diagnosis

The differential diagnosis for catheter-related complications includes the following conditions:

An exit site infection refers to an infection localized to the area where the catheter exits the skin, indicating a potential source of microbial invasion at the catheter insertion site. Phlebitis, characterized by the inflammation of a vein, often manifests with symptoms such as pain, redness, and swelling along the affected vein, highlighting the vascular inflammatory response triggered by the catheter. Pocket infections, which occur in the subcutaneous pocket where the catheter is implanted, can lead to localized abscess formation and tissue damage due to microbial proliferation in the implantation site.

Sepsis, a severe systemic infection, can arise from the dissemination of microorganisms from the catheter into the bloodstream, causing a life-threatening condition necessitating urgent intervention to prevent septic shock and multiple organ dysfunction. Tunnel infection denotes an infection along the tunnel created during catheter insertion, typically following the path of the catheter, indicating a potential breach in aseptic technique during the insertion procedure. Urinary tract infection (UTI) may be considered in cases where symptoms overlap with catheter-related issues, warranting evaluation for concurrent urinary tract involvement and potential microbial colonization associated with catheter use. Each of these diagnostic entities presents with distinct clinical features, necessitating a thorough evaluation to differentiate between them accurately, enabling the implementation of tailored diagnostic and therapeutic strategies to address the specific underlying pathology.

The precise identification of the causative factor is paramount for initiating appropriate management protocols aimed at resolving the catheter-related complication effectively and preventing further complications or systemic sequelae. In conclusion, a comprehensive understanding of the differential diagnosis for catheter-related complications is essential for healthcare providers to deliver optimal patient care and ensure positive clinical outcomes in individuals with indwelling catheters.

4.20 Prevention Guidelines During Insertion

1. Hand hygiene, which involves the practice of washing hands with soap, water, or alcohol-based gel, is an essential measure to prevent the spread of infections in healthcare settings. It is crucial to understand that gloves are not a substitute for proper hand hygiene and should be used in conjunction with handwashing practices. When it comes to maintaining strict aseptic technique during procedures such as central venous catheter insertion, healthcare providers should adhere to maximal sterile barrier precautions. This includes the use of a full-body drape to minimize the risk of contamination and reduce the chances of introducing pathogens into the patient's bloodstream.
2. To further enhance infection control measures, the employment of a 2% chlorhexidine solution for disinfecting or cleaning the skin before catheter insertion is highly recommended. This practice has been shown to effectively reduce the risk of infections associated with central venous catheters. Additionally, the use of ultrasound guidance for catheter placement, under the supervision of an experienced provider, is essential in preventing mechanical complications and reducing the number of insertion attempts required. Vein selection is another critical aspect to consider, with the femoral vein being avoided for central line placement whenever possible. Instead, the subclavian vein is preferred for non-tunneled catheters due to a lower risk of complications.
3. In cases where a central line is no longer necessary, it is imperative to promptly remove it to minimize the risk of infections and other associated complications. Central lines that were inserted during emergency situations, where asepsis may not have been ensured, should be replaced as soon as possible or within 48 h to reduce the risk of infections. Implementation of a checklist during central line placement is a valuable tool to ensure that all essential steps and precautions are followed. This systematic approach helps in reducing errors and complications, ultimately improving patient safety and outcomes in healthcare settings.

4.21 Prevention Guidelines During Maintenance

1. Before gaining access to the line, it is crucial to meticulously disinfect the catheter hubs, injection ports, and connections to reduce the likelihood of contamination and subsequent infection. This step is essential in maintaining a safe

healthcare environment and minimizing the risks associated with invasive procedures. Moreover, by adhering to strict disinfection protocols, healthcare providers can effectively safeguard patients from potentially harmful pathogens.

2. Furthermore, the replacement of administration sets, with the exception of those designated for lipids or blood products, should occur every 96 h. This routine practice plays a pivotal role in preventing the buildup of microbial colonies and upholding a state of asepsis throughout the duration of intravenous therapy. Timely replacement of administration sets is essential for ensuring the delivery of safe and effective care to patients.
3. In addition to catheter hub disinfection and administration set replacement, daily assessment of central lines is recommended. This daily evaluation serves as a proactive measure to determine the ongoing necessity of the central line, thereby reducing the chances of unnecessary exposure and potential complications associated with prolonged catheter use. Healthcare providers must prioritize regular assessments to uphold patient safety and quality of care.
4. Consequently, by implementing these best practices, healthcare facilities can enhance patient outcomes, reduce the incidence of healthcare-associated infections, and promote a culture of safety and excellence in clinical practice. Adherence to these guidelines is essential for mitigating risks and ensuring optimal patient care. It is imperative that healthcare professionals remain vigilant in their commitment to following established protocols for catheter care and maintenance.

4.22 Summary

Catheter-related bloodstream infection (CRBSI) is a healthcare-acquired problem that results in significant morbidity, mortality, extended hospitalizations, and escalated expenditures. In order to address CRBSI, it is essential to develop local guidelines that prioritize the daily assessment of the requirement for the Central Venous Catheter (CVC) and the enforcement of a proactive approach to promptly remove it when deemed unnecessary. The proactive measures are vital for averting complications linked to prolonged catheterization and play a pivotal role in enhancing patient outcomes and optimizing resource allocation within healthcare settings. By implementing these strategies, healthcare facilities can effectively combat CRBSI and enhance the quality of care provided to patients.

References

1. Hallam C, Jackson T, Rajgopal A, Russell B. Establishing catheter-related bloodstream infection surveillance to drive improvement. J Infect Prev. 2018;19(4):160–6.
2. Aloush SM, Alsaraireh FA. Nurses' compliance with central line-associated bloodstream infection prevention guidelines. Saudi Med J. 2018;39(3):273–9.

3. Gaholt R, Nigam C, et al. Catheter-related bloodstream infections. Int J Crit Illn Inj Sci. 2014;4(2):162–7.
4. Chopdekar K, Chande C, Chavan S, Veer P, Wabale V, Vishwakarma K, Joshi A. Central venous catheter-related blood stream infection rate in critical care units in a tertiary care, teaching hospital in Mumbai Central venous catheter-related blood stream infection rate in critical care units in a tertiary care, teaching hospital in Mumbai. Indian J Med Microbiol. 2011;29(2):169–71.
5. Singh S, Pandya Y, Patel R, Paliwal M, Wilson A, Trivedi S. Surveillance of device-associated infections at a teaching hospital in rural Gujarat—India. IJMM. 2010;28(4):342–7.
6. Parameswaran R, Sherchan JB, Varma DM, Mukhopadhyay C, Vidyasagar S. Intravascular catheter-related infections in an Indian tertiary care hospital. J Infect Dev Ctries. 2011;5:452–8.
7. Maki DG, Kluger DM, Crnich CJ. The risk of bloodstream infection in adults with different intravascular devices: a systematic review of 200 published prospective studies. Mayo Clin Proc. 2006;81:1159–71.
8. Soufir L, Timsit JF, Mahe C, Carlet J, Regnier B, Chevret S. Attributable morbidity and mortality of catheter-related septicemia in critically ill patients: a matched, risk-adjusted, cohort study. Infect Control Hosp Epidemiol. 1999;20:396–401.
9. Pronovost P, Needham D, Berenholtz S, Sinopoli D, Chu H, Cosgrove S, et al. An intervention to decrease catheter-related bloodstream infections in the ICU. N Engl J Med. 2006;355:2725–32.
10. Cicaline S, Palmieri F, Petrosillo N. Clinical review: new technologies for prevention of intravascular catheter-related infections. Crit Care. 2004;8:157–62.
11. Lee H, Manns B, Taub K, Ghali WA, Dean S, Johnson D, et al. Cost analysis of ongoing care of patients with end-stage renal disease: the impact of dialysis modality and dialysis access. Am J Kidney Dis. 2002;40:611–22.
12. Bouza E, Alvarado N, Alcala L, et al. A prospective, randomized, and comparative study of 3 different methods for the diagnosis of intravascular catheter colonization. Clin Infect Dis. 2005;40:1096–100.
13. Mermel LA, McCormick RD, Springman SR, Maki DG. The pathogenesis and epidemiology of catheter-related infection with pulmonary artery Swan-Ganz catheters: a prospective study utilizing molecular subtyping. Am J Med. 1991;91:197S–205.
14. Powe NR, Jaar B, Furth SL, Hermann J, Briggs W. Septicemia in dialysis patients incidence, risk factors, and prognosis. Kidney Int. 1999;55:1081–90.
15. Garland JS, Buck RK, Maloney P, Durkin DM, Toth-Llyod S, Duffy M, et al. Comparison of 10% povidone-iodine and 0.5% chlorhexidine gluconate for the prevention of peripheral intravenous catheter colonization in neonates: a prospective trial. Pediatr Infect Dis J. 1995;14:510–6.
16. Sachdev A, Gupta D, Soni A, Chugh K. Central venous catheter colonization and related bacteremia in pediatric intensive care unit. Indian Pediatr. 2002;39:752–60.
17. Gopalakrishnan R, Sureshkumar D. Changing trends in antimicrobial susceptibility and hospital acquired infections over an 8 year period in a tertiary care hospital in relation to introduction of an infection control programme. J Assoc Physicians India. 2010;58(Suppl):25–31.
18. Seifert H, Cornely O, Seggewiss K, Decker M, Stefanik D, Wisplinghoff H. Bloodstream infection in neutropenic cancer patients related to short-term nontunnelled catheters determined by quantitative blood cultures, differential time to positivity, and molecular epidemiological typing with pulsed-field gel electrophoresis. s. 2003;41:118–23.
19. Almuneef MA, Memish ZA, Balkhy HH, Hijazi O, Cunningham G, Francis C. Rate, risk factors and outcomes of catheter related bloodstream infection in a paediatric intensive care unit in Saudi Arabia. J Hosp Infect. 2006;62:207–13.
20. Pawar M, Mehta Y, Kapoor P, Sharma J, Gupta A, Trehan N. Central venous catheter-related blood stream infections: incidence, risk factors, outcome, and associated pathogens. J Cardiothorac Vasc Anesth. 2004;18:304–8.

21. Allon M. Dialysis catheter-related bacteremia: treatment and prophylaxis. Am J Kidney Dis. 2004;44:779–91.
22. Nassar GM, Ayus JC. Infectious complications of the hemodialysis access. Kidney Int. 2000;60:1–13.
23. Beathard GA. Management of bacteremia associated with tunneled-cuffed hemodialysis catheters. J Am Soc Nephrol. 1999;10:1045–9.
24. Kovalik EC, et al. A clustering of epidural abscesses in chronic hemodialysis patients: risks of salvaging access catheters in cases of infection. J Am Soc Nephrol. 1996;7:2264–7.
25. Maki DG, Weise CE, Sarafin HW. A semiquantitative culture method for identifying intravenous-catheter-related infection. N Engl J Med. 1977;296:1305–9.
26. Brun-Buisson C, Abrouk F, Legrand P, Huet Y, Larabi S, Rapin M. Diagnosis of central venous catheter-related sepsis—critical level of quantitative tip cultures. Arch Intern Med. 1987;147:873–7.
27. Bouza E, Alvarado N, Alcala L, Perez MJ, Rincon C, Munoz P. A randomized and prospective study of 3 procedures for the diagnosis of catheter-related bloodstream infection without catheter withdrawal. Clin Infect Dis. 2007;44:820–6.
28. Wilcox MH, Tack KJ, Bouza E, et al. Complicated skin and skin structure infections and catheter-related bloodstream infections: noninferiority of linezolid in a phase 3 study. Clin Infect Dis. 2009;48:203–12.
29. Reboli AC, Rotstein C, Pappas PG, et al. Anidulafungin versus fluconazole for invasive candidiasis. N Engl J Med. 2007;356:2472–82.
30. Fernandez-Hidalgo N, Almirante B, Calleja R, Ruiz I, Planes AM, Rodriguez D, et al. Antibiotic-lock therapy for long-term intravascular catheter-related bacteraemia: results of an open, non-comparative study. J Antimicrob Chemother. 2006;57:1172–80.
31. Raad I, Davis S, Khan A, Tarrand J, Elting L, Bodey GP. Impact of central venous catheter removal on the recurrence of catheter-related coagulase-negative staphylococcal bacteremia. Infect Control Hosp Epidemiol. 1992;13:215–21.
32. Chopdekar K, Chande C, Chavan S, Veer P, Wabale V, Vishwakarma K, Joshi A. Central venous catheter-related blood stream infection rate in critical care units in a tertiary care, teaching hospital in Mumbai. Indian J Med Microbiol. 2011;29(2):169–71.
33. Pawar M, Mehta Y, Purohit A, Trehan N, Daniel RV. Resistance in gram-negative bacilli in a cardiac intensive care unit in India: risk factors and outcome. Ann Card Anaesth. 2008;11(1):20–6.

Chapter 5
Catheter-Associated Urinary Tract Infections (CAUTI): Prevalence and Management

5.1 CAUTI: Prevention and Management

Hospital-acquired infections (HAI) represent a significant issue in healthcare settings, often leading to prolonged hospital stays and complications arising from the use of medical devices and improper patient care practices. Among the various types of HAI, those associated with invasive devices such as central lines, catheters, and ventilators are particularly prevalent. Central line-associated bloodstream infections, catheter-associated urinary tract infections, and ventilator-associated pneumonia are among the most commonly reported HAIs related to invasive devices [1]. It is worth noting that a substantial proportion of these infections are attributed to multidrug-resistant organisms, posing a serious challenge to treatment. In the realm of HAI, catheter-associated urinary tract infections (CAUTI) stand out as a major concern, accounting for a significant percentage of all UTIs occurring during hospitalizations. Specifically, it has been reported that around 80% of UTIs in hospitalized patients are linked to the use of indwelling urethral catheters. The clinical implications of CAUTI, which may include conditions such as prostatitis, pyelonephritis, and cystitis, are particularly worrisome within the intensive care unit (ICU) setting, where patients are already vulnerable to various complications. As such, effective strategies for preventing and managing CAUTI are crucial in improving patient outcomes and reducing the burden of HAI in healthcare facilities.

5.2 CAUTI (CDC Definition)

A urinary tract infection (UTI) is defined as an infection that occurs when a urinary catheter has been in place for over two consecutive days at the time of the occurrence, with the initial day of catheter insertion considered as Day 1. The presence of

R. Chakraverty, A. K. Kundu, *Hospital-Acquired Infections in Intensive Care Unit and their Management*, https://doi.org/10.1007/978-981-96-0018-2_5

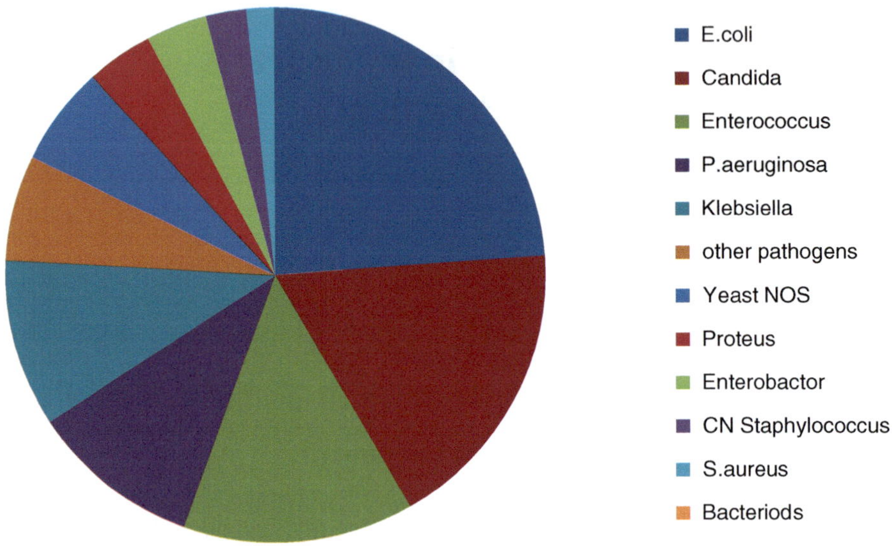

Fig. 5.1 Pie chart showing causative organism of CAUTI

an indwelling urinary catheter either on the day of the event or the preceding day is crucial for the categorization of a UTI. In cases where an indwelling urinary catheter has been present for more than two calendar days and is subsequently removed, the date of the UTI event should be recorded as the day of catheter removal or the following day in order to establish a catheter-associated UTI.

5.3 Causative Organism of CAUTI

The following pie chart shows causative organism of CAUTI as shown in Fig. 5.1.

5.4 Risk Factor of CAUTI

1. *Gender*: Females are more prone to catheter-associated infection.
2. *Age*: Geriatric group of patients admitted in hospital with other chronic illness or other site of infection have greater risk of infections than younger age of people.
3. *Period of catheterization*: The longer period of catheterization, specifically for more than 10 days, unchanged urinary bag, and unchanged urinary tube all are risk factors of CAUTI.
4. *Diabetes mellitus, immunocompromised* patients are at more risk for CAUTI.

5. *Patients with renal insufficiency* are more prone to infections.
6. Patients with *neurological deficits* are more at risk for CAUTI.

5.5 Impact of CAUTI

1. The prolonged duration of hospitalization can be attributed to various factors such as the complexity of the medical condition, the need for extensive treatment protocols, and the occurrence of complications during the patient's stay in the healthcare facility.
2. The rise in morbidity rates and mortality outcomes can be linked to a range of interconnected variables including the severity of the illness, the presence of underlying health issues, and the effectiveness of the medical interventions provided to the patients.
3. The escalation in hospital expenses is a multifaceted issue influenced by factors such as the utilization of advanced medical technologies, the cost of pharmaceuticals, the length of hospital stays, and the intensity of care required by patients with critical health conditions.
4. The surge in antimicrobial usage within healthcare settings is a critical concern due to its implications on the development of antimicrobial resistance, the potential for adverse drug reactions, and the financial burden associated with the procurement of antimicrobial agents to combat infectious diseases.

5.6 Pathogenesis of CAUTI [2]

The origin of microorganisms can either stem from within the body (such as colonization in the urethra, rectum, or vagina) or from external sources, typically introduced through the unsterile hands of healthcare workers while inserting catheters or handling urinary collection systems. This transmission can lead to infections in patients, highlighting the importance of proper hand hygiene and aseptic techniques in healthcare settings.

5.7 CAUTI Diagnostic Pathway

Signs and Symptoms of CAUTI

1. Fever/rigor/altered mental status without alternative explanation
2. Flank pain, costovertebral angle tenderness
3. Acute hematuria
4. Patient with chronic spinal cord injury with worsening spasticity or autonomic dysreflexia

5.8 Modified HICPAC Categorization Scheme for Recommendations as Shown in Table 5.1

Table 5.1 Showing modified HICPAC categorization scheme for recommendations

Category 1A	A robust recommendation backed by substantial to moderate quality evidence indicating clear clinical advantages or disadvantages is crucial in guiding healthcare decisions
Category 1B	Such recommendations can greatly influence patient outcomes and the overall quality of care provided
Category 1C	On the contrary, a weak recommendation supported by evidence of any quality may indicate a delicate balance between clinical benefits and potential harms, requiring careful consideration by healthcare professionals
Category II	Additionally, unresolved issues characterized by low to very low-quality evidence present challenges in assessing the trade-offs between benefits and harms, posing dilemmas for clinicians and policymakers alike
No recommendation/ unresolved issue	Furthermore, a well-established practice upheld by scanty evidence of low to very low quality may be deemed acceptable in certain scenarios, shedding light on the complexities of evidence-based medicine. Lastly, compliance with state or federal regulations may necessitate a strong recommendation, underscoring the intersection of evidence-based guidelines and legal mandates in healthcare decision-making processes

5.9 Prevention Strategy of CAUTI

Core strategies encompass approaches that are founded on high levels of scientific evidence, which serve as the cornerstone for effective implementation and outcomes in various fields. The robust foundation of high scientific evidence not only ensures the validity and reliability of the strategies but also enhances their credibility and potential impact on the target audience. Demonstrated feasibility is another crucial aspect of core strategy, indicating that these approaches have been tested and proven to be viable, practical, and implementable in real-world settings. The demonstration of feasibility provides stakeholders with the assurance that the strategies can be successfully executed and integrated into existing systems or practices.

In addition to core strategies, supplemental strategies play a significant role in expanding the range and effectiveness of prevention efforts. While these strategies may have varying levels of scientific evidence supporting them, they offer valuable complementary approaches to address specific aspects or challenges within a prevention framework. Similarly, the feasibility of supplemental strategies may vary, with some exhibiting high levels of practicality and applicability, while others may require further testing or adaptation for successful implementation.

Core prevention strategies, classified as Category 1B interventions, represent a set of fundamental principles and practices that are universally recommended for preventing infections associated with catheter use. These strategies include inserting catheters only when clinically indicated, ensuring timely removal of catheters, and restricting catheter insertion and maintenance to trained personnel. Moreover, adherence to aseptic techniques and sterile equipment during catheter insertion is essential to minimize the risk of infections.

Following aseptic insertion, maintaining a closed drainage system and unobstructed urine flow are critical components of catheter care that help prevent contamination and blockages. Additionally, promoting hand hygiene practices and standard precautions, or implementing appropriate isolation measures when necessary, further enhance infection control efforts in healthcare settings. By adhering to these core prevention strategies, healthcare providers can significantly reduce the incidence of catheter-associated infections and improve patient outcomes.

5.9.1 Core Prevention Strategies

5.9.1.1 Specific Recommendations (Ib)

Example of Appropriate Indications for Indwelling Urethral Catheter Use

1. In patients experiencing acute urinary retention or obstruction at the bladder outlet, there is a critical need for precise measurement of urinary output, especially in those who are critically ill. This is particularly critical in the perioperative environment, especially for specific surgical procedures such as those involving the genitourinary tract or urologic structures. Additionally, in situations where the operation is predicted to last a long time, a tube might be placed, and it must be promptly taken out in the post-anesthesia care unit (PACU) to avoid issues. Additionally, patients who are expected to receive large volumes of infusions or diuretics during the surgical procedure necessitate accurate monitoring of urine output intraoperatively. Moreover, in instances where there is a need to facilitate the healing process of open sacral and perineal wounds in patients with incontinence, measuring urinary output is crucial. For patients requiring extended periods of immobilization, such as those with unstable thoracic or lumbar spine injuries, monitoring urine output is vital to prevent urinary retention. Lastly, in end-of-life care scenarios, accurate measurement of urinary output can also contribute to improving the comfort and overall quality of care for patients if required.

Minimize the utilization of catheters in all patients, especially those who are at a heightened risk of developing catheter-associated urinary tract infections (CAUTI) and experiencing mortality. It is imperative to exercise caution when considering the use of catheters for the management of incontinence. Catheters should only be employed in operative patients when deemed absolutely necessary to their treatment.

Furthermore, it is vital to ensure that catheters are only retained for the duration required for their intended purpose. Postoperative removal of catheters should be prioritized, ideally within a 24-h timeframe following the procedure, unless there exist valid reasons to prolong their use.

During the insertion of catheters in acute care settings, practitioners should adhere strictly to aseptic techniques and utilize sterile equipment. Hand hygiene practices should be rigorously observed both before and after the insertion procedure. Additionally, special attention should be given to minimizing catheter usage, particularly in patients with heightened susceptibility to CAUTI and mortality, and refraining from using catheters for incontinence management. Moreover, the practice of leaving catheters in place for only the necessary duration is crucial to prevent complications. Postoperatively, catheters should be promptly removed, preferably within the first 24 h, unless there are specific clinical indications necessitating their continued presence.

When inserting catheters, it is essential to follow strict aseptic techniques and use sterile equipment to minimize the risk of infections. Proper hand hygiene practices should be observed before and after the insertion procedure. Additionally, sterile gloves, drapes, sponges, antiseptic solutions, or sterile solutions should be used for periurethral cleaning, and catheters should be adequately secured post-insertion. Following the aseptic insertion of catheters, maintaining a closed drainage system is crucial to prevent infections. In cases where breaches in aseptic technique, disconnections, or leakages occur, the catheter and collecting system should be replaced using sterile equipment and aseptic techniques. Consideration should be given to utilizing systems with preconnected, sealed catheter tubing junctions, and urine samples should be obtained aseptically for testing purposes.

To ensure unobstructed urine flow, it is essential to keep the catheter and collecting tube free from kinks and ensure that the collecting bag remains positioned below the level of the bladder at all times. Regular emptying of the collecting bag using separate, clean containers for each patient is necessary, and precautions should be taken to prevent the drainage spigot from coming into contact with nonsterile surfaces.

Instituting quality improvement programs is essential to promote the appropriate use of indwelling catheters and reduce the risk of CAUTI. Examples of such programs include implementing alerts or reminders, utilizing stop orders, establishing protocols for nurse-directed catheter removal, and developing guidelines for perioperative catheter management.

5.9.2 Supplemental Prevention Strategies [3]

The first example pertains to the exploration of alternatives to the insertion of indwelling urinary catheters. One such strategy involves employing portable ultrasound devices for the purpose of evaluating urine volume, which can effectively contribute to a reduction in unnecessary catheterizations. Additionally, another approach involves utilizing catheters that are impregnated with antimicrobial or antiseptic agents, thereby potentially mitigating the risk of infections. Moreover, intermittent catheterization should be taken into consideration for specific patient populations, such as those necessitating chronic urinary drainage due to conditions like neurogenic bladder resulting from spinal cord injuries, myelomeningocele in children, or postoperative patients experiencing urinary retention. This method may also be employed in conjunction with a bladder ultrasound scanner for enhanced efficacy. Furthermore, external catheters may be deemed suitable for cooperative male patients who do not have any obstruction or issues with urinary retention. Lastly, the utilization of bladder ultrasound scanners has been shown to have a positive impact by reducing the frequency of catheterizations, consequently leading to a decrease in catheter-associated urinary tract infections (CAUTI). Similarly, the utilization of silver-coated catheters has demonstrated a decreased risk of bacteriuria when compared to standard latex catheters.

5.10 Strategies Not Recommended for CAUTI Prevention

The urinary drainage system can be quite intricate due to its complexity, involving various components and mechanisms to ensure proper functioning and drainage of urine. One common practice is the regular changing of catheters or drainage bags at specific, predetermined intervals to prevent complications such as infections or blockages. This routine maintenance is essential in maintaining the integrity of the system and promoting optimal urinary health. Another common practice is the use of routine antimicrobial prophylaxis, which involves the administration of antibiotics to prevent urinary tract infections or other complications associated with catheter use.

Furthermore, it is crucial to emphasize the importance of cleaning the periurethral area with antiseptic solutions while the catheter is in place to reduce the risk of contamination and infection. This meticulous cleaning process helps to maintain a sterile environment and minimize the chances of introducing harmful pathogens into the urinary tract. Additionally, the irrigation of the bladder with antimicrobial solutions can be beneficial in reducing bacterial growth and preventing infections that may arise from stagnant urine.

Moreover, the instillation of antiseptic and antimicrobial solutions in the drainage bag is a common practice to further inhibit bacterial growth and maintain a clean and sterile environment within the system. This proactive approach to infection prevention can significantly reduce the incidence of catheter-related complications and promote better patient outcomes. Routine screening for asymptomatic bacteriuria is also recommended to detect any potential infections early on and initiate appropriate treatment promptly to prevent further complications.

In conclusion, the management of a complex urinary drainage system requires a multifaceted approach that includes regular maintenance, prophylactic measures, meticulous cleaning procedures, and proactive infection prevention strategies. By adhering to these practices, healthcare providers can help minimize the risks associated with urinary catheterization and promote better urinary health outcomes for patients.

5.11 Measurement: Example of Process Measures

Compliance with hand hygiene is essential in healthcare settings to prevent the spread of infections and ensure patient safety. It is crucial for healthcare workers to adhere to proper hand hygiene protocols, such as washing hands with soap and water or using hand sanitizer before and after patient contact, to reduce the risk of transmitting harmful microorganisms. Additionally, compliance with an educational program focusing on hand hygiene practices can further reinforce the importance of this infection control measure among healthcare staff. Furthermore, documenting the insertion and removal of catheters, as well as indicating the reasons for catheter placement, is vital for maintaining accurate patient records and monitoring the appropriateness of catheter use in clinical practice. Compliance with these documentation requirements can contribute to improving patient outcomes and reducing healthcare-associated infections.

5.12 Measurement: Recommended Outcome Measures

The metrics are as follows:

1. Number of CAUTI per 1000 catheter days
2. Number of BSI secondary to CAUTI per 1000 catheter days
3. Catheter utilization ratio (urinary catheter days/patient days) ×100

5.13 Treatment of CAUTI

5.13.1 Empiric Treatment for CAUTI

Drug of choice for mild to moderate CAUTI

1. Ciprofloxacin 500 mg po or 400 mg IV q 12 h
2. Levofloxacin 500–750 mg IV/po q 24 h
3. Ceftriaxone 1 g IV daily

Drug of choice in severe CAUTI

1. Cefepime 2 g IV q 12 h
2. Ceftazidime 2 g IV q 8 h
3. Imipenem 500 mg IV q 6 h
4. Meropenem 1 g q 8 h
5. Piperacillin–tazobactam 3.375–4.5 g IV q 6 h.
   Dose adjustment may be necessary in reduced renal function.

5.13.2 Catheter Irrigation

A comprehensive review conducted by the Cochrane collaboration meticulously examined the existing body of evidence pertaining to the practice of catheter irrigation/washout as a preventive measure against blockage and infection in individuals with indwelling catheters. The analysis, which scrutinized a total of seven trials, highlighted that the quality of these trials was notably subpar and presented limitations in their methodology [4]. Consequently, the review authors concluded that the available evidence did not reach a substantial level to offer concrete recommendations concerning the potential benefits and risks associated with catheter washout. Notably, the trials under review exhibited heterogeneity in their approach, utilizing varying irrigation solutions ranging from saline to acidic solutions, as well as implementing different protocols.

Subsequent to this review, a randomized controlled clinical trial involving 60 comatose patients in intensive care units provided further insights into the efficacy of daily bladder irrigation with normal saline in reducing the risk of catheter-associated urinary tract infections (CAUTIs). While this trial yielded promising results, the overall evidence supporting the use of gentamicin or betadine irrigation for the prevention of urinary tract infections (UTIs) remains limited [5]. For instance, findings from a retrospective study indicated that intravesical administration of gentamicin led to a reduction in symptomatic UTI episodes, oral antibiotic usage, and the prevalence of antibiotic-resistant organisms [6]. Moreover, another study illustrated that daily intravesical irrigation of the bladder with povidone-iodine was linked to a significant decrease in symptomatic UTIs among patients with neurogenic bladder and recurrent UTIs who underwent clean intermittent catheterization. However, to validate these preliminary findings and ascertain their applicability to individuals with indwelling catheters, further randomized clinical trials are imperative. These trials must be designed to provide robust evidence on the efficacy and safety of different catheter irrigation methods, thereby enhancing our understanding of the optimal strategies for UTI prevention in this patient population.

5.13.3 Asymptomatic Bacteriuria

Current guidelines currently discourage the practice of screening for or providing treatment for asymptomatic bacteriuria, a condition characterized by the presence of bacteria in the urine without any signs of infection. However, it is important to note that there are two significant exceptions to this recommendation. The first exception pertains to pregnant individuals, as the presence of asymptomatic bacteriuria in this population has been associated with an increased risk of developing symptomatic urinary tract infections (UTIs) and other complications during pregnancy. The second exception applies to individuals who are scheduled to undergo urologic surgery that carries a risk of mucosal trauma or manipulation of the upper urinary tract, as addressing asymptomatic bacteriuria prior to the procedure can help reduce the likelihood of postoperative infections [7].

Specifically, the Infectious Diseases Society of America (IDSA) provides guidance against the screening for or treatment of asymptomatic bacteriuria in individuals with spinal cord injury, as well as those with short-term (lasting less than 30 days) or long-term indwelling catheters. This recommendation is based on the understanding that asymptomatic bacteriuria in these populations is often a benign condition that does not necessarily require intervention, and treating it with antibiotics can lead to the development of antimicrobial resistance and other adverse effects. Similarly, the guidelines from the American Urological Association (AUA) also discourage the treatment of asymptomatic bacteriuria, aligning with the stance taken by the IDSA. It is essential to acknowledge that the clinical presentation of UTIs in individuals with spinal cord injury or other neurologic conditions may differ from those without such underlying pathologies. Due to the altered neurogenic bladder function and sensory deficits commonly observed in these patients, the typical signs and symptoms of UTIs may be subtle or atypical [8]. Therefore, healthcare providers caring for this population must exercise caution and attentiveness in evaluating any potential indicators of UTI, as a high level of suspicion is necessary to promptly diagnose and manage these infections in individuals with neurologic impairments.

5.13.4 Prevention and Challenges

Despite the measures mentioned above, catheter-associated urinary tract infections (CAUTIs) persist as a prevalent issue with significant economic implications. The rise in antibiotic resistance poses a growing concern, a matter acknowledged by the World Health Organization, labeling it as one of the most substantial threats to global public health. This recognition is further emphasized by the acknowledgment of antibiotic usage as a major contributing factor to this escalating problem [9]. Furthermore, the unintended consequences of antibiotic administration include the disruption of the balance of the healthy gut microbiome, leading to potential issues such as pathogen proliferation and the translocation of harmful toxins. Consequently, there is a pressing need to explore alternatives to conventional antibiotics [10]. This necessity has sparked a surge of interest in non-antibiotic strategies aimed at preventing CAUTIs. The ensuing section delves into the various opportunities available for the prevention of CAUTIs at different stages of development and clinical evaluation [11].

5.14 Conclusion

Catheter-associated urinary tract infections (CAUTIs) represent the most common healthcare-associated infection and are the primary cause of secondary bloodstream infections, characterized by alarmingly high levels of resistance to antibiotics. The diagnosis of CAUTIs entails the examination of urine culture results and evaluation of symptoms, tasks that pose difficulties and are subjects of debate, especially for patients with indwelling catheters. Novel preventive strategies encompass a range of approaches including the development of catheter coatings, novel materials, and vaccines. Among the promising avenues for prevention is the concept of bacterial interference, which involves the introduction of nonpathogenic microbial strains to competitively inhibit the growth of harmful pathogens in the urinary tract, thereby diminishing the risk of CAUTIs. Advancements in diagnostic methodologies and tools to aid in treatment decisions are currently underway, incorporating various biomarkers often combined with cutting-edge technologies like artificial intelligence and the analysis of cell-free DNA, among others. Despite the challenges faced by the current antibiotic research and development pipeline in keeping up with the pace of resistance evolution, recent approvals by the FDA have been granted for new medications designed to combat multidrug resistant complicated urinary tract infections. Research efforts are also exploring alternative treatments to conventional antibiotics, including inhibitors that target specific mechanisms involved in bacterial pathogenesis, such as the assembly of adhesive pili that facilitate adherence to catheters and the bladder. These inhibitors, referred to as mannosides and pilicides, are engineered to disrupt pathogenic processes without impacting essential metabolic pathways, thereby sidestepping the development of antibiotic resistance and minimizing effects on the healthy gut and vaginal microbiota. These innovative strategies hold great promise and significance in the context of the escalating threat of antibiotic resistance. Ongoing investigations across clinical, translational, and fundamental scientific domains are continuously enriching our comprehension and approach toward the management of CAUTIs. Acknowledging the substantial hurdles encountered in this field and harnessing the existing body of knowledge will undoubtedly play a pivotal role in shaping the future landscape of CAUTI management.

References

1. Flores-Mireles A, Hreha TN, Hunstad DA. Pathophysiology, treatment, and prevention of catheter-associated urinary tract infection. Top Spinal Cord Inj Rehabil. 2019;25(3):228–40.
2. Gould CV, Umscheid CA, Agarwal RK, Kuntz G, Pegues DA, Healthcare Infection Control Practices Advisory Committee. Guideline for prevention of catheter-associated urinary tract infections 2009. Infect Control Hosp Epidemiol. 2010;31(4):319–26.
3. Popovich KJ, Calfee DP, Patel PK, Lassiter S, Rolle AJ, Hung L, Saint S, Chopra V. The Centers for Disease Control and Prevention STRIVE initiative: construction of a national program to reduce health care–associated infections at the local level. Ann Intern Med. 2019;171(7_Suppl):S2–6.
4. Shepherd AJ, Mackay WG, Hagen S. Washout policies in long-term indwelling urinary catheterisation in adults. Cochrane Database Syst Rev. 2017;(3):CD004012. https://doi.org/10.1002/14651858.CD004012.

5. Ramezani F, Khatiban M, Rahimbashar F, Soltanian AR. Efficacy of bladder irrigation in preventing urinary tract infections associated with short-term catheterization in comatose patients: a randomized controlled clinical trial. Am J Infect Control. 2018;46(10):e45–50. https://doi.org/10.1016/j.ajic.2018.05.009.
6. Cox L, He C, Bevins J, Clemens JQ, Stoffel JT, Cameron AP. Gentamicin bladder instillations decrease symptomatic urinary tract infections in neurogenic bladder patients on intermittent catheterization. Can Urol Assoc J. 2017;11(9):E350. https://doi.org/10.5489/cuaj.4434.
7. Gould CV, Umscheid CA, Agarwal RK, Kuntz G, Pegues DA, Healthcare Infection Control Practices Advisory Committee. Guideline for prevention of catheter-associated urinary tract infections 2009. Infect Control Hosp Epidemiol. 2010;31(4):319–26. https://doi.org/10.1086/651091.
8. Bagley K, Severud L. Preventing catheter-associated urinary tract infections with incontinence management alternatives: pureWick and condom catheter. Nurs Clin. 2021;56(3):413–25. https://doi.org/10.1016/j.cnur.2021.05.002.
9. Fakih MG, Watson SR, Greene MT, et al. Reducing inappropriate urinary catheter use: a statewide effort. Arch Intern Med. 2012;172(3):255–60. https://doi.org/10.1001/archinternmed.2011.627.
10. Rosenthal V, Todi S, Alvarez-Moreno C, et al. Impact of a multidimensional infection control strategy on catheter-associated urinary tract infection rates in the adult intensive care units of 15 developing countries: findings of the International Nosocomial Infection Control Consortium (INICC). Infection. 2012;40(5):517–26. https://doi.org/10.1007/s15010-012-0278-x.
11. Saint S, Greene MT, Kowalski CP, Watson SR, Hofer TP, Krein SL. Preventing catheter-associated urinary tract infection in the United States: a national comparative study. JAMA Intern Med. 2013;173(10):874–9. https://doi.org/10.1001/jamainternmed.2013.101.

Chapter 6
Surgical Site Infections (SSI): Prevalence and Management

6.1 Introduction

Surgical site infections (SSIs) are the most prevalent and expensive hospital-acquired infections, constituting 20% of all HAIs. It is noted that SSIs occur in 2–5% of patients who undergo in-patient surgery, leading to an extended hospital stay averaging 9 days and a mortality rate that is 2–11 times higher. The infections themselves are responsible for almost 77% of these fatalities. The prescription of perioperative antimicrobials is commonly observed in healthcare settings. The Centers for Disease Control and Prevention's [1–4] National Healthcare Safety Network (NHSN) categorizes SSIs based on the depth and tissues affected: superficial SSI involves only the skin or subcutaneous tissue, deep incisional SSI affects the fascia and/or muscular layers, and organ space SSI involves any part of the body opened or manipulated during a procedure excluding the aforementioned layers. Surgical site infections (SSIs) are associated with prolonged hospitalization, death, and poor overall patient outcomes. SSIs are usually caused by pathogens inoculated from the patient's own plant at the time of surgery. The acquisition of SSI depends on the host's capacity to be exposed to bacteria and control the inevitable bacterial contamination of the surgical wound. The nine core best practices for reducing SSIs include preoperative bathing, antimicrobial prophylaxis, and preoperative surgical sites. Surgery site infection (SSI) is an infection that occurs in an invasive surgical procedure that causes the incision. SSI is the main cause of hospital morbidity and has prolonged hospital stays, increased hospital costs, increased reoperation costs, and even higher mortality rates. Primary management is prevention through good surgical techniques and patient optimization. The SSI rate varies depending on the type of surgery, and with the worsening of the level of contamination, the rate increases. SSIs can be classified according to the tissue: superficial SSI = limited to skin and subcutaneous tissues, deep SSI = affects fascial and muscular layers, cavity space infection = in the abdomen or joint cavity.

R. Chakraverty, A. K. Kundu, *Hospital-Acquired Infections in Intensive Care Unit and their Management*, https://doi.org/10.1007/978-981-96-0018-2_6

6.2 Epidemiology

Surgical site infections (SSIs) represent the most prevalent and financially burdensome healthcare-associated infection (HAI) within the borders of the United States, constituting nearly a quarter of all HAIs [5]. The incidence of SSIs remains relatively modest; however, their prevalence is significant due to the substantial number of surgical interventions conducted nationwide. Notably, in the year 2014, a staggering 17.2 million hospital visits, encompassing both outpatient and inpatient settings, involved invasive and therapeutic surgical procedures. Statistics indicate that SSIs develop in approximately 1–5% of individuals undergoing inpatient surgeries, with rates generally exhibiting a downward trend among various surgical interventions [6].

6.3 Clinical Outcomes

Surgical site infections (SSIs) result in considerable patient morbidity and mortality, posing a serious threat to postoperative recovery. It has been reported that each incidence of SSI prolongs the hospital stay by an estimated 7–11 days, highlighting the impact of these infections on healthcare resources and patient well-being. Collectively, patients affected by SSIs contribute to an alarming 3.7 million surplus hospital days annually, underscoring the urgency for effective prevention and management strategies. Furthermore, individuals who develop SSIs following surgery face a mortality risk that is notably higher, ranging from 2-fold to 11-fold compared to those who do not experience such complications, with a substantial 77% of SSI-related deaths being directly linked to the infection itself [7–9].

6.4 Evaluation

Clinically speaking, a surgical incision is classified as infected when there is the presence of purulent drainage at the site of the cut or when there are indications of an abscess forming in the surgical area. Nonetheless, there are also other manifestations of infections in surgical wounds that can manifest, such as wound dehiscence, drainage that is not purulent, localized redness, hardening of the tissue, discomfort, or signs of a systemic infection. Due to the diverse array of ways in which surgical site infections can present themselves, some of which may be similar to symptoms caused by noninfectious factors, there is no singular clinical definition that encapsulates all SSIs. Consequently, healthcare professionals must remain vigilant and consider various factors when assessing the possibility of a surgical wound infection [10].

6.5 Current Evidence (Table 6.1)

Surgical site infections (SSIs) commonly result from the introduction of pathogens during the surgical procedure. The majority of SSIs are attributed to the patient's own flora, originating from within the body. Nonetheless, it is also plausible for external sources to contaminate the surgical wound. Skin pathogens are the primary culprits behind most SSIs, although gastrointestinal procedures may introduce enteric pathogens into the mix. Among the various pathogens, *S. aureus* stands out as the predominant agent responsible for causing SSIs. Historically, methicillin-resistant *S. aureus* (MRSA) held a higher prevalence in SSIs compared to methicillin-sensitive strains (MSSA); however, recent trends indicate a shift in MRSA rates [12].

Table 6.1 Showing operation, likely pathogens, and antibiotic use prophylactically before surgery [11]

Operation	Likely pathogen	Prophylactic antibiotic before surgery
Placement of all grafts, prostheses, or implants	*Staphylococcus aureus*; CoNS	Cefazoline or cefuroxime
Cardiac	*Staphylococcus aureus*; CoNS	Cefazoline or cefuroxime
Neurosurgery	*Staphylococcus aureus*; CoNS	Cefazoline or cefuroxime
Breast	*Staphylococcus aureus*; CoNS	Cefazoline or cefuroxime
Ophthalmic	*S. aureus*; CoNS; streptococci; gram-negative bacilli	Moxifloxacin given as one drop every 5–15 min for five doses
Orthopedic total joint replacement, closed fractures/use of nails, bone plates, other internal fixation devices, functional repair without implant/device	*Staphylococcus aureus*; CoNS; gram-negative bacilli	Cefazolin For 'below-the-belt' surgeries, piperacillin-tazobactam + clindamycin
Noncardiac thoracic (lobectomy, pneumonectomy wedge resection, other noncardiac mediastinal procedures), closed tube thoracostomy	*Staphylococcus aureus*; CoNS; gram-negative bacilli	Cefazoline or cefuroxime or ampicillin-sulbactam
Vascular	*Staphylococcus aureus*; CoNS	Cefazolin or cefuroxime
Appendectomy	gram-negative bacilli	Piperacillin-tazobactam

6.6 Guidelines for Prevention [13]

Several detailed published guidelines for SSI prevention exist, including the following four published primary guideline documents:

1. The document titled "Strategies to Prevent Surgical Site Infections in Acute Care Hospitals: 2014 Update" was sponsored by the Society for Healthcare Epidemiology of America (SHEA), with contributions from members of various other organizations well-versed in the field of surgical site infection prevention. This collaborative effort signifies the importance of different stakeholders coming together to address the critical issue of surgical site infections in acute care settings.
2. The involvement of multiple organizations with expertise in SSI prevention underscores the comprehensive nature of the guidelines put forth in the document, aiming to provide healthcare facilities with a robust framework for reducing the incidence of surgical site infections and improving patient outcomes. Similarly, the World Health Organization (WHO) has issued "Global Guidelines for the Prevention of Surgical Site Infection," emphasizing the global impact of surgical site infections and the need for a unified approach to preventing such infections across different healthcare settings worldwide.

6.7 Therapeutic Options

Surgical debridement and excision of the infected tissue stands out as the paramount aspect of treatment for numerous surgical site infections (SSIs), while the administration of antimicrobial therapy serves as a crucial supplementary element. It is imperative to note that the specific method of debridement and the duration of antimicrobial treatment hinge on factors such as the extent of the infection, the location within the body, and the presence of prosthetic devices. Nonetheless, it is universally acknowledged that infections classified as deep-incisional or involving organ/space typically necessitate surgical removal of the infected tissue through operative means.

6.8 Assessment

The Study of the Efficacy of Nosocomial Infection Control (SENIC) was carried out by the CDC in order to assess the cost-effectiveness of various infection prevention activities, which also included surveillance. Numerous studies, including the SENIC study, have consistently demonstrated that infection surveillance programs and providing feedback on surgical site infection (SSI) rates to surgeons can lead to a significant decrease in overall SSI rates ranging from 32 to 50%. These findings have played a crucial role in shaping the CDC's recommendation that hospitals should regularly conduct surveillance for SSIs and share this information for reporting purposes.

6.9 Summary

Surgical site infections (SSIs) are prevalent and expensive healthcare-related infections within the United States, resulting in substantial patient morbidity and mortality. It is crucial to follow evidence-based preventive measures to reduce the incidence of SSIs. Generally, the treatment of SSI involves a combination of aggressive surgical debridement and the administration of suitable antibiotic therapy to ensure successful management of the infection.

References

1. Enoch D, Whitney L. Antimicrobial Stewardship from principles to practice. Birmingham: British Society of Antimicrobial Chemotherapy; 2018.
2. Global guidelines for the prevention of surgical site infection. World Health Organization; 2018.
3. Allegranzi B, Bagheri Nejad S, Combescure C, Graafmans W, Attar H, Donaldson L, et al. Burden of endemic health-care-associated infection in developing countries: systematic review and meta-analysis. Lancet. 2011;377(9761):228–41.
4. Mangram AJ, Horan TC, Pearson ML, Silver LC, Jarvis WR, Hospital Infection Control Practices Advisory Committee. Guideline for prevention of surgical site infection, 1999. Infect Control Hosp Epidemiol. 1999;20(4):247–80.
5. Anderson DJ, Podgorny K, Berrios-Torres SI, Bratzler DW, Dellinger EP, Greene L, Nyquist AC, Saiman L, Yokoe DS, Maragakis LL, Kaye KS. Strategies to prevent surgical site infections in acute care hospitals: 2014 update. Infect Control Hosp Epidemiol. 2014;35(S2):S66–88.
6. Van Kasteren ME, Mannien J, Kullberg BJ, de Boer AS, Nagelkerke NJ, Ridderhof M, Wille JC, Gyssens IC. Quality improvement of surgical prophylaxis in Dutch hospitals: evaluation of a multi-site intervention by time series analysis. J Antimicrob Chemother. 2005;56(6):1094–102.
7. Gouvêa M, Novaes CD, Pereira DM, Iglesias AC. Adherence to guidelines for surgical antibiotic prophylaxis: a review. Braz J Infect Dis. 2015;19(5):517–24.
8. https://www.cdc.gov/hai/ssi/ssi.html. Accessed 7 Jan 2021.
9. https://www.cdc.gov/nhsn/pdfs/pscmanual/17pscnosinfdef_current.pdf. Accessed 11 Jan 2021.
10. Protocol for surgical site infection surveillance with a focus on settings with limited resources. Geneva: World Health Organization; 2018. Licence: CC BY-NC-SA 3.0 IGO.
11. Antibiotic policy IPGMER 2023.
12. Berríos-Torres SI, Umscheid CA, Bratzler DW, Leas B, Stone EC, Kelz RR, Reinke CE, Morgan S, Solomkin JS, Mazuski JE, Dellinger EP. Centers for disease control and prevention guideline for the prevention of surgical site infection, 2017. JAMA Surg. 2017;152(8):784–91.
13. Brink AJ, Messina AP, Feldman C, Richards GA, van den Bergh D, Netcare Antimicrobial Stewardship Study Alliance. From guidelines to practice: a pharmacist-driven prospective audit and feedback improvement model for peri-operative antibiotic prophylaxis in 34 South African hospitals. J Antimicrob Chemother. 2017;72(4):1227–34.

Chapter 7
Surgical Antimicrobial Prophylaxis (SAP) in India

7.1 Introduction

Surgical site infection (SSI) is a term utilized to encompass infections in both the surgical wound and infections affecting the body cavity and organs, which may or may not be linked to implants or prosthetic devices [1]. The administration of antibiotics as a preventive measure serves to inhibit the growth of contaminating bacteria and their adherence to prosthetic implants, thereby reducing the likelihood of infection. The World Health Organization's (WHO) Clean Care is Safer Care program has demonstrated that SSI is the most common type of hospital-acquired infection (HAI) in low-middle-income countries (LMICs), impacting up to one-third of patients who have undergone a surgical procedure. In LMICs, the combined incidence rate of SSI was 11.8 per 100 surgical procedures, with a range from 1.2 to 23.6. Despite the fact that the incidence of SSI is significantly lower in high-income countries, it still remains the second most prevalent type of HAI [2]. Even though SSI is considered one of the most preventable HAIs, it continues to pose a substantial burden in terms of patient morbidity and mortality, as well as incurring additional costs for health systems and service payers on a global scale [3].

The most cost-effective intervention that should be implemented in the healthcare setting, according to the guidelines provided by the World Health Organization for the prevention of surgical site infections (SSI), is the prevention of SSI. It has been reported that at least 60% of SSI occurrences could be prevented by the implementation of best practices. The implementation of the best infection prevention practices and the appropriate use of surgical antimicrobial prophylaxis (SAP) are the most proven methods of infection prevention and control. However, there has been an observed trend of overdependence on antimicrobials for the prevention of infections, leading to their inappropriate use, which can have detrimental consequences [4].

R. Chakraverty, A. K. Kundu, *Hospital-Acquired Infections in Intensive Care Unit and their Management*, https://doi.org/10.1007/978-981-96-0018-2_7

The inappropriate use of SAPs, such as prolonged duration and the use of broad-spectrum antibiotics, has the potential to select resistant microorganisms, thereby resulting in high costs. Furthermore, incorrect timing of prophylaxis can reduce its efficacy. Consequently, the quality of prophylaxis has been the subject of numerous audits and intervention studies, leading to the development of guidelines by national and interventional bodies to support its correct use. Despite the clearly established principles of SAPs and their proven effectiveness, global adherence to these guidelines is generally poor. Recent reviews and studies have highlighted noncompliance in up to 88% of surgical cases, indicating a significant gap in practice [5].

The reasons for nonadherence to guidelines appear to be complex and multifactorial, encompassing factors such as fears of litigation, lack of clinician awareness of updated guidelines, absence of enforceable policies, and failures in the implementation of institutional norms, guidelines, and patient care systems. It is essential to monitor the appropriateness of prescriptions for SAP to determine if prescribing aligns with best practices. Auditing serves as a valuable starting point to provide baseline information and to identify areas where changes are needed for improvement. Measures should be established to capture data during auditing, which can then be utilized to monitor the success of the changes implemented.

7.2 Objectives [6]

1. In order to explore the realm of surgical antimicrobial prophylaxis (SAP), in addition to preventive measures adopted by patients undergoing surgeries with a clean contaminated classification, one must delve into the estimation of the surgical site infection (SSI) incidence and the subsequent identification of risk factors that are closely linked with SSI occurrence.
2. Furthermore, it is imperative to uncover the obstacles hindering the execution of effective surgical prophylaxis practices and to strategize on the creation and execution of a comprehensive set of antimicrobial stewardship (AMS) interventions, which may include educational initiatives and training sessions, as well as prospective audit and feedback mechanisms, all aimed at enhancing SAP.
3. This approach aims to evaluate the effectiveness of these interventions in reducing the incidence of SSI, thus shedding light on the impact of such interventions on overall surgical outcomes.

7.3 Methodology

1. Study design:
   Settings: Multicentric prospective intervention study.

2. Patient population:
   Patients who are scheduled to undergo clean-contaminated wound surgery within the timeframe tentatively set between February 2021 to September 2021 at the designated research locations will be included in the research study. Clean-contaminated wound surgeries encompass operative wounds where entry into the respiratory, alimentary, genital, or urinary tracts occurs under controlled circumstances and without any exceptional contamination, assuming there is no indication of infection or significant deviation in technique. Exclusion criteria will apply to patients who are unable to communicate independently or may prove challenging to reach post-surgery due to unavoidable circumstances arising [7].

   In the context of this study, a surgical site infection is defined as an infection that emerges following a surgical procedure in the specific area of the body where the surgery was performed. These infections can range from superficial ones affecting solely the skin to more severe cases involving tissues beneath the skin, organs, or any implanted material. The calculation of SSI events for reporting purposes will involve considering all patients who underwent the chosen operative procedure/s at the research site for SSI monitoring during the study period as the denominator.

On the other hand, the numerator for SSI event reporting will comprise all patients who underwent the selected operative procedure/s at the research site and subsequently develop an SSI, which encompasses superficial incisional SSI, deep incisional SSI, or organ/space SSI within a 1-month surveillance timeframe. The diagnosis and classification of SSI will adhere to the criteria established by the Centers for Disease Control and Prevention (CDC). These criteria serve as the standard for identifying and categorizing SSI cases, ensuring consistency and accuracy in reporting and analysis.

7.3.1 Duration of Study

The study work plan shall have three phases.

Phase I: During the pre-implementation phase lasting for a duration of 2 months, a comprehensive period is dedicated to laying the groundwork for the subsequent steps in the implementation process. This initial stage involves meticulous planning, analysis, and preparation to ensure a smooth transition into the intervention phase. Following this preparatory period, an additional 2 weeks are allocated for conducting a thorough survey aimed at identifying potential obstacles and challenges that may impede the successful implementation of surgical prophylaxis measures.

Phase II: Subsequently, a period of 2 months is designated for the detailed planning and execution of the intervention, which primarily focuses on education and training initiatives. This phase entails the development of tailored strategies and resources to effectively educate and train relevant stakeholders on the importance and application of surgical prophylaxis measures. Moreover, the implementation of these measures is meticulously planned and executed to ensure maximum efficacy and adherence.

Phase III: Following the intervention phase, a post-implementation period spanning over 4 months is dedicated to monitoring and evaluating the outcomes through the implementation of Prospective audit and feedback mechanisms. This critical phase involves the systematic assessment of the effectiveness of the implemented measures, gathering feedback from stakeholders, and making necessary adjustments to optimize the outcomes. Continuous monitoring and feedback mechanisms are essential components of this phase to ensure sustained improvements in surgical prophylaxis practices [8].

So total duration of study will be of 8 months and 2 weeks.

7.3.2 Sample Size and Sampling Strategy

This study is designed as a before and after intervention study, aiming to enhance the process outcome, specifically the quality of prophylaxis. The methodology chosen for participant selection is the purposive sampling method, ensuring that patients meeting the eligibility criteria and undergoing the designated surgery at each center during the study period will be included in the research. The decision to employ purposive sampling is strategic, as it allows for a targeted approach to participant selection, aligning with the study's primary objective of improving prophylaxis quality.

The preliminary findings from a point prevalent survey conducted previously revealed a high percentage of inappropriate surgical prophylaxis, specifically in terms of duration, with a rate of 86%. This indicates a significant area for improvement. By setting a goal to reduce this percentage to 68% with a power of 90%, the calculated sample size required is 110. Therefore, to achieve this target and ensure robust results, the total sample size for the study is set at 500 participants. This translates to 100 participants per center, allocated evenly between the pre-implementation and post-implementation phases of the study.

The meticulous planning of sample size allocation for each phase of the study is crucial for obtaining reliable and generalizable results. By enrolling a substantial number of participants from each center, the study aims to capture a comprehensive picture of the impact of the intervention on prophylaxis quality. The division of participants into pre- and post-implementation groups allows for a direct comparison of outcomes, enabling a clear assessment of the intervention's effectiveness.

The strategic distribution of participants across different phases and centers enhances the study's internal validity, minimizing potential biases and confounding factors. Additionally, the large sample size increases the study's statistical power, enabling the detection of smaller yet clinically significant differences in prophylaxis quality. This approach not only strengthens the study's scientific rigor but also enhances its ability to contribute valuable insights to the field of surgical prophylaxis.

In conclusion, the careful selection of the purposive sampling method and the meticulous planning of sample size allocation are essential components of this before and after intervention study. By setting clear objectives, defining precise sample size requirements, and strategically dividing participants, the study aims to generate robust evidence on the impact of the intervention on improving the quality of surgical prophylaxis.

7.3.3 Information Sheets and Consent

The study, which entails the collection of data based on records, poses minimal risk, thus prompting the center to formally petition the ethics committee for a possible exemption from obtaining consent. Should this exemption not be granted, it will be imperative to secure written informed consent from all patients participating in the study, a practice that ensures ethical standards are upheld. In addition to this, patients will receive detailed information sheets outlining the purpose and procedures of the study, fostering transparency and understanding among participants.

Furthermore, patients can rest assured that their identities will remain anonymous throughout the data collection process, safeguarding their privacy and confidentiality. Similarly, healthcare professionals involved in the surgical procedures will also be guaranteed anonymity in the overall reporting of the study findings. To maintain confidentiality, any reports specific to surgeons or units will be encoded, thus preventing the inclusion of personal identifiers or information that could compromise privacy. It is crucial to underscore that regardless of a patient's involvement in the study, there will be no disparities in the treatment or care they receive, ensuring equity and quality healthcare for all individuals.

7.3.4 Study Procedure [9]

This will be a prospective multicentric intervention study.

A training session will be conducted by the lead center on data collection. Following this, a pilot run for each committed surgical procedure will be conducted for at least five surgical procedures by participating centers within 2 weeks. A follow-up meeting will be conducted by the lead center. Any suggestions or modifications in the proposed plan will be discussed at this point. A training session led by the main center on data collection will be conducted, followed by a pilot run for each committed surgical procedure to be carried out by the participating center. This pilot run will encompass at least five surgical procedures within a timeframe of 2 weeks. Subsequently, a follow-up meeting will be organized by the lead center where any suggestions or modifications to the proposed plan will be thoroughly deliberated.

During Phase I of the study, which focuses on perioperative data collection, pertinent details of the patient will be inputted into the data collection form (Annexure I; Part-I). This information will include demographic specifics of the patient, details on preoperative and intraoperative preventive measures, information on perioperative antimicrobial usage, type of surgery, ASA score, duration of surgery, and details on other risk factors associated with the development of surgical site infections (SSI). Part II of the form will encompass information on postoperative follow-up details and any occurrences of SSI.

The adapted WHO perioperative data collection form10 will be utilized throughout the study, both in Phase I and Phase III (pre- and post-implementation period). Each surgical procedure will necessitate the completion of a perioperative data collection form. Efforts will be made to extract all necessary details from the patients' clinical records. In cases where information is missing, or further details are required, the attending healthcare professional will be consulted. The aim is to complete the pre- and intraoperative details within 48 h of the surgery.

Regarding postoperative follow-up, the study will focus on monitoring patients for up to 30 days post-operation (with the day of the operation being considered as day 1) to detect any potential development of SSI. This will involve follow-ups with patients in the clinic after hospital discharge or via telephonic consultations where face-to-face visits are not feasible.

Throughout the 30-day period, a total of three patient reviews are planned, approximately at the end of week 1, week 2, and week 4 post-operation. However, there is a commitment to ensure at least one postoperative interaction with the patient after discharge, either through a clinical visit or via a telephonic conversation if necessary. If there are five unsuccessful attempts to reach a patient by telephone, they will be considered lost to follow-up. The primary goal is to achieve complete follow-up on more than 90% of patients under surveillance.

During postoperative visits, the wound will be examined by a specialist from the respective clinical discipline, and the patient's history of antibiotic treatment will be documented. In cases of telephonic contact, a structured interview will be conducted to identify any SSIs (refer to Annexure II). If there are suspicions of an SSI, the patient will be advised to visit the hospital for direct visualization of the wound by the relevant clinician. If this is not feasible, the patient will be referred to the nearest healthcare facility.

The responsible clinician will be tasked with diagnosing and classifying any SSIs based on CDC definitions [10, 11].

Details about the patients gathered from their case records during inpatient or outpatient encounters, as well as information obtained through telephone interactions, will be documented in the perioperative data collection form. The comprehensive data collection process ensures that all relevant information pertaining to the patients' medical history and current status is accurately captured for clinical decision-making purposes. This meticulous approach to data collection plays a crucial role in enhancing the quality of patient care and optimizing outcomes in both inpatient and outpatient settings.

If any one or all of the following is inappropriate, it would be considered inappropriate surgical prophylaxis practice.

1. Choice of antimicrobial
2. Dose of antimicrobial
3. Timing of administration of the antimicrobial
4. Duration of administration of the antimicrobial

In order to determine the suitability of the aforementioned actions, a consensus framework will be formulated to outline the recommended procedures for the surgeries to be included, drawing from the directives established by the Nodal Center, RD Gardi Medical College, ICMR, and NCDC. This crucial process will be executed through the organization of a virtual assembly involving all the primary investigators and co-investigators within the collective. The assessment of the infection prevention and control (IPC) methods will be conducted in alignment with the guidelines provided by the Centers for Disease Control and Prevention for the prevention of surgical site infections, as outlined in the comprehensive document released in 2017 [9].

7.3.4.1 Assessment of Barriers in Implementing Correct Surgical Prophylaxis Practices

A survey instrument designed to evaluate the obstacles will be created to identify the hindrances to the execution of surgical preventive measures. It will be distributed to 30 surgeons at each facility. The design of the survey will be influenced by the prior experiences of these facilities. Each facility will aim to include surgeons from various specialties and levels of experience. The results of the surveys conducted with surgeons, as well as those examining surgical site infections (SSI), will inform the development of an intervention strategy.

7.3.4.2 Phase II: Education and Training

A team of surgeons who partook in the survey will be assembled. There will be the utilization of two training modules: (1) A specialized 2-h session (one-time occurrence) and (2) an ongoing small-group, local feedback, and training program that will span the final 4 months.

Following the analysis of the initial phase's results, a virtual 2-h program will be carried out. This program will encompass: (1) The dissemination of data from the SSI survey and obstacles to implementation, (2) deliberation on best practices, and (3) a panel discussion involving surgeons esteemed as exemplars of appropriate surgical prophylaxis procedures.

A small booklet of good surgical prophylaxis practices will be developed and shared in all the centers.

Each individual center will formulate a detailed plan aimed at overcoming the obstacles that have been identified within their specific locations. For example, in cases where it has been determined that the fear of breaches in infection control protocols is driving the excessive use of antimicrobials, it will be imperative to collaborate closely with the infection control team at the respective hospitals in order to devise and execute appropriate strategies. Similarly, if the root cause is found to be a fundamental gap in comprehension regarding prophylaxis principles, it will be necessary to organize intimate local group discussions, ideally with the participation of a local influencer, to address this issue. These targeted interventions at the center level are crucial for ensuring effective and sustainable improvements in healthcare practices and outcomes.

Phase III: Post-implementation with prospective audit and feedback entails the utilization of a perioperative data collection form (Annexure I) for the evaluation of adherence to preventive measures' practices and the suitability of the selection of AMA, dose, timing, and redoing. Following this initial phase, a review and feedback process will be carried out. Two types of feedback mechanisms will be implemented. One will be on an individual case basis, while the other will be on a group basis. Individual case feedback will be delivered through telephonic messages, emails, or in-person communication. On the other hand, group feedback will follow the same approach as previously used in the nodal center, where departmental faculty members are gathered, and the antimicrobial stewardship team conducts discussions and addresses relevant issues. At least two sessions of such feedback will be conducted locally within a span of 4 months.

7.3.5 *Measuring the Impact of the AMS Practices: Process and Outcome Indicators [12]*

No.	Measure	Indicator
Process measures		
1.	The appropriateness of the chosen antibiotic for a particular medical procedure depends on various factors such as the type of infection, the susceptibility of the causative organism, the patient's medical history, and the potential for drug interactions or adverse effects. In order to determine whether the antibiotic choice was appropriate, it is essential to consider all of these factors in conjunction with current clinical guidelines and best practices in antimicrobial stewardship	Rate of adherence to the antibiotic selection in relation to the type of surgery or the use of a substitute agent[a]
2.	Was the antibiotic dosage administered at the appropriate level as prescribed?	Rate of adherence to the antibiotic dosage or adherence to weight-based dosing when recommended[b]

(continued)

No.	Measure	Indicator
3.	Was the antibiotic administered within a 60-min window before the commencement of the surgical procedure?[c]	Compliance rate within 60 min with the administration
4.	Antibiotic duration[d]:	Compliance with the single dose is monitored, or, if applicable, re-dosed[d] or discontinued within 24 h after the beginning of the operation
	(a) Was the antibiotic administered in a singular dosage?	
	(b) Was the antibiotic readministered if deemed necessary?	
	(c) Was the antibiotic administered for a duration exceeding 24 h?	
Outcome measures		
5	The number of SSIs occurring postoperatively	SSI rate[e]

[a]In patients with β-lactam allergies, was the chosen alternative appropriate?
[b]In case of cefazolin, gentamicin, and vancomycin, was weight-based dosing used complaint with the guideline?
[c]Administration within 120 min of incision for vancomycin and fluoroquinolones
[d]Redosing acceptable for cases of intraoperative blood loss >1500 mL or procedures greater than 2.5 h long
[e]SSI rate: For the computation of the rate of surgical site infections (SSI), the denominator refers to the total count of patients who have received the specific operative procedure/s designated by the research site within the defined study period. In the numerator for SSI event documentation, it encompasses patients who experience SSI incidents (encompassing superficial incisional SSI, deep incisional SSI, or organ/space SSI) over a duration of 1 month during the surveillance period

The process measure indicators encompass the suitability of the selection of AMA, dosage, timing, and duration. The standardized measurements will be determined as ratios in relation to the quantity of surgical patients observed by the surveillance team, where the denominator is the total number of patients participating in the research and the numerator represents those who adhere to each of the four process indicators.

Overall compliance with the four process measures will be calculated as follows:

The sum of the total number of indicators with which the doctors are compliant/ divided by the total number of indicators (n/4).

Outcome measure: SSIs occurring postoperatively will be recorded independently by the surveillance team according to standard CDC definition and classification [10, 11]. For feasibility reasons, SSI occurring within 30 days of operation will be considered.

SSI rates per 100 operative procedures will be calculated by dividing the number of SSIs by the number of surgical procedures audited and multiplying the result by 100. Improvements in compliance with the prophylaxis bundle will be measured.

7.3.6 *Data Management and Analysis*

All the information will be documented on a predetermined case record form (Annexure I). This form will be transformed into an Epi-info format suitable for utilization on a tablet. The various centers will distribute the spreadsheets produced by this format with the primary center on a weekly basis. Each principal investigator will randomly authenticate 25% of the information.

The data from each center and the compiled data will undergo a process of data scrubbing. Following the resolution of any inquiries, the data will be finalized and examined. Summary statistics featuring measures of variability for both categorical and continuous data, as appropriate, will be produced. The surgical site infection (SSI) rate will be computed as the ratio of SSI occurrences to every 100 procedures. The percentages of adherence to individual performance indicators for processes and the total compliance with the four process indicators will be computed as previously mentioned. Comparisons in compliance and SSI rates between the phases before and after the intervention will be conducted utilizing the chi-square test. A significance level of $p < 0.05$ will be deemed noteworthy.

References

1. Enoch D, Whitney L. Antimicrobial Stewardship from principles to practice. Birmingham: British Society of Antimicrobial Chemotherapy; 2018.
2. Global guidelines for the prevention of surgical site infection. World Health Organization; 2018.
3. Allegranzi B, Bagheri Nejad S, Combescure C, Graafmans W, Attar H, Donaldson L, et al. Burden of endemic health-care-associated infection in developing countries: systematic review and meta-analysis. Lancet. 2011;377(9761):228–41.
4. Mangram AJ, Horan TC, Pearson ML, Silver LC, Jarvis WR, Hospital Infection Control Practices Advisory Committee. Guideline for prevention of surgical site infection, 1999. Infect Control Hosp Epidemiol. 1999;20(4):247–80.
5. Anderson DJ, Podgorny K, Berrios-Torres SI, Bratzler DW, Dellinger EP, Greene L, Nyquist AC, Saiman L, Yokoe DS, Maragakis LL, Kaye KS. Strategies to prevent surgical site infections in acute care hospitals: 2014 update. Infect Control Hosp Epidemiol. 2014;35(S2):S66–88.
6. Van Kasteren ME, Mannien J, Kullberg BJ, de Boer AS, Nagelkerke NJ, Ridderhof M, Wille JC, Gyssens IC. Quality improvement of surgical prophylaxis in Dutch hospitals: evaluation of a multi-site intervention by time series analysis. J Antimicrob Chemother. 2005;56(6):1094–102.
7. Gouvêa M, Novaes CD, Pereira DM, Iglesias AC. Adherence to guidelines for surgical antibiotic prophylaxis: a review. Braz J Infect Dis. 2015;19(5):517–24.
8. Protocol for surgical site infection surveillance with a focus on settings with limited resources. Geneva: World Health Organization; 2018. Licence: CC BY-NC-SA 3.0 IGO.
9. Berríos-Torres SI, Umscheid CA, Bratzler DW, Leas B, Stone EC, Kelz RR, Reinke CE, Morgan S, Solomkin JS, Mazuski JE, Dellinger EP. Centers for disease control and prevention guideline for the prevention of surgical site infection, 2017. JAMA Surg. 2017;152(8):784–91.
10. https://www.cdc.gov/hai/ssi/ssi.html. Accessed 7 Jan 2021.
11. https://www.cdc.gov/nhsn/pdfs/pscmanual/17pscnosinfdef_current.pdf. Accessed 11 Jan 2021.
12. Brink AJ, Messina AP, Feldman C, Richards GA, van den Bergh D, Netcare Antimicrobial Stewardship Study Alliance. From guidelines to practice: a pharmacist-driven prospective audit and feedback improvement model for peri-operative antibiotic prophylaxis in 34 South African hospitals. J Antimicrob Chemother. 2017;72(4):1227–34.

Chapter 8
Antimicrobial Stewardship Practices in Intensive Care Units in India

8.1 Introduction

Antimicrobial resistance (AMR) represents a substantial global menace to public health and advancement, leading to extended hospitalizations, heightened medical costs, and elevated fatality rates. It impacts individuals of all age brackets and influences diverse sectors such as healthcare, veterinary medicine, and agriculture, thus emerging as a critical global health issue. The surge of AMR places in jeopardy the bedrock of contemporary medicine and weakens the efficacy of worldwide public health strategies against infectious ailments. In the absence of prompt and united action on a global scale, there is a looming risk of entering a post-antibiotic era where common infections reemerge as life-threatening challenges [1].

India emerges as the foremost consumer of antibiotics for human use globally, with an astonishing annual consumption rate of 12.9×10^9 units. The economic ramifications of AMR, encompassing healthcare expenditures and reduced productivity, are significant, with the United States registering an annual burden of $55 billion and global forecasts projecting losses amounting to $100 trillion by 2050 if unaddressed. Alarmingly, up to 90% of the anticipated ten million deaths linked to AMR are anticipated to transpire in low-and middle-income nations (LMICs), underscoring the immediate necessity for interventions in these regions [2–5].

Acknowledging the severity of the situation, the Indian Council of Medical Research (ICMR) initiated the Antimicrobial Resistance Surveillance and Research Network (AMRSN) in 2013, aligning with international endeavors to combat AMR, as delineated in the Chennai Declaration. In 2017, the National Health Policy of India accorded precedence to AMR, culminating in the inception of the National Action Plan on AMR in April 2017, with the objective of addressing AMR and advocating for responsible antibiotic utilization throughout healthcare domains.

This section seeks to assess the efficacy of antimicrobial stewardship programs (ASPs) executed in India based on available literature. These initiatives are

R. Chakraverty, A. K. Kundu, *Hospital-Acquired Infections in Intensive Care Unit and their Management*, https://doi.org/10.1007/978-981-96-0018-2_8

formulated to enhance the management of infections, diminish infection-related morbidity and mortality, curb the emergence of multidrug-resistant organisms (MDROs), and curtail unnecessary antimicrobial usage. Effective ASPs ensure the judicious choice, dosage, and duration of antimicrobials, thereby ameliorating clinical outcomes while mitigating adverse effects. They additionally oversee prescription patterns, enforce regulations to rationalize antibiotic usage, and aid in minimizing the detrimental repercussions of antibiotics. Over the past decade, AMSP has been validated by multiple studies to foster appropriate antimicrobial use, mitigate AMR and its dissemination, enhance patient results, and reduce healthcare costs. Consequently, AMSP has gained traction in numerous countries and regions. Nations such as Australia, Chile, China, France, Scotland, South Africa, South Korea, Sweden, Taiwan, the United States, and Vietnam have effectively implemented antibiotic stewardship initiatives. Stewardship programs are extensively adopted in the United States, where compliance with various guidelines is assessed annually through the National Healthcare Safety Network Annual Hospital Survey [6, 7].

In tertiary hospitals in China, the establishment of an antimicrobial stewardship program has been examined to identify the potential challenges for the AMSP and to offer references and benchmarks for strategic policymaking, as discussed [8]. The escalation of drug resistance in pathogens of public health significance has led to a crisis situation globally, including in India. Hospitals in India have been reporting significant levels of resistance to fluoroquinolones and carbapenems, and the escalating trends of antibiotic resistance in the country are concerning, particularly with the rising percentage of resistance to last-resort antibiotics such as carbapenems and colistins, as highlighted [9] and the ICMR annual report (2019).

The capacities of AMSPs in Indian healthcare institutions (HCIs) are basic or even nonexistent, a fact well-documented in a survey conducted by ICMR in 2013 among 20 tertiary HCIs, focusing on AMSP components, implementation, and outcomes [2, 10]. The survey revealed that only 40% of HCIs possessed written AMSP documents, 75% had HIC guidelines, and 65% had AMAs prescription guidelines. Process measures are the most straightforward to assess, as they use proxy indicators to show whether an AMSP has effectively altered processes (e.g., adherence to guidelines/clinical pathways), prescriber behavior (e.g., accurate diagnosis, appropriate drug-indication pairing, correct antimicrobial dosage, frequency, and duration, as well as appropriate and timely therapeutic adjustments) [11–13]. Despite being relatively easy to collect and providing valuable data, process measures alone are insufficient for achieving objectives such as optimizing antimicrobial selection (i.e., drug, dose, and duration) and reducing adverse drug events (e.g., morbidity, mortality, length of hospital stay, and healthcare costs). Both process and outcome measures are crucial components of any quality improvement initiative and should be integrated into the hospital's antimicrobial stewardship plan. Interventions aimed at evaluating process and/or outcome measures for monitoring and reporting antimicrobial usage and outcomes data are vital not only for assessing the effectiveness of the AMSP but also for identifying areas for enhancement, according to CDC (2014).

Therefore, by concentrating on evaluating process and outcome measures linked to AMSPs in all 20 tertiary care hospitals within the ICMR AMR network, this study will ensure precise and consistent data collection on antibiotic utilization, aiding in optimizing antimicrobial selection and reducing adverse drug events in our hospital. Furthermore, only 30% of HCIs had AMSP implementation strategies in place. Private HCIs exhibited better performance in AMSP compared to government HCIs, with this disparity being attributed to the accreditation process. This disparity highlights a gap in AMSP implementation in India, emphasizing the urgent need to prioritize the implementation of AMSPs [14]. Recognizing the necessity to establish AMSP structures in HCIs across the country, the ICMR conducted four workshops on AMSP capacity building nationwide in the second quarter of 2017. The website (http://iamrsn.icmr.org.in/index.php/events/amsp) has been utilized for hosting various events related to the AMSP program, and a range of efforts have been put in place to enhance the capabilities of individuals as well as to allocate financial resources to ensure the successful execution and continuity of the AMSP program within tertiary care hospitals starting from the year 2018 [15].

8.2 Infection Encountered in Critical Care Units

One encounters a maximum combination of community-acquired and healthcare-associated infections (HAIs) in critical care areas due to a variety of factors such as prolonged length of stay, presence of comorbidities and complex health conditions, utilization of invasive procedures and devices, and the critical condition of patients, among others. It is crucial to differentiate between community-acquired and healthcare-associated infections as the causative agents and their susceptibility patterns differ significantly. Understanding the types of microorganisms expected to be present aids in the selection of appropriate empiric antibiotics and facilitates decisions regarding the escalation or de-escalation of antibiotic therapy. The co-occurrence of community-acquired and healthcare-associated infections in critical care settings can be attributed to several factors including extended length of hospital stays, presence of underlying health conditions, utilization of invasive medical procedures and devices, as well as the critical state of patients. Distinguishing between community-acquired and healthcare-associated infections is essential due to the distinct nature of the causative agents and their susceptibility profiles. Knowledge of the anticipated microorganisms is valuable for selecting appropriate empiric antibiotics and guiding decisions on antibiotic escalation or de-escalation [16].

The selection of antibiotics should ideally be guided by organizational policies that consider the susceptibility patterns of prevalent microorganisms in each healthcare facility. In order to promote consistency and encourage antimicrobial stewardship, a national guideline for syndrome-based antimicrobial treatment was introduced in 2016 and subsequently updated in the following year. This guideline was developed by consolidating susceptibility data from major healthcare institutions nationwide. In addition to adhering to guideline-based antibiotic choices, healthcare providers can also refer to institutional antibiotic policies that reflect local antibiogram data. These guidelines and policies play a crucial role in mitigating the risk of antimicrobial resistance by limiting the use of broad-spectrum antibiotics. Furthermore, they support the judicious use of antibiotics among junior medical staff and private practitioners, contributing to overall antimicrobial stewardship efforts [17–20].

8.3 AMR in Healthcare

A most recent global report released by the World Health Organization (WHO) in April 2019 has brought to light the alarming AMR crisis that is currently unfolding across the globe. According to the report, the projected mortality rate due to infections resistant to multiple drugs is estimated to reach a staggering ten million deaths annually by the year 2050, a significant increase from the current annual death toll of 700,000. These projected statistics underscore the urgent need for immediate interventions to address the looming global threat posed by AMR. The escalating trend of drug resistance among a variety of organisms is a cause for growing concern. The misuse and abuse of antimicrobial agents have played a pivotal role in fueling the spread of AMR, exacerbating the crisis at hand. An optimal antimicrobial prescription should adhere to the principle of administering the "right drug at the right dose and right time through the right route for the right duration." The development of antimicrobial resistance occurs when this fundamental principle is violated, coupled with inadequate infection control measures, leading to the proliferation and dissemination of multidrug-resistant microorganisms [21, 22]. Furthermore, a significant drawback of antimicrobial usage is the phenomenon known as "collateral damage," which pertains to the detrimental impact on the normal microbiota inhabiting the human body. The gastrointestinal tract, for instance, harbors trillions of beneficial microorganisms that play critical roles in maintaining health through various mechanisms. These include the secretion of essential vitamins such as K and B12, competition with pathogens for attachment sites and nutrients, production of antimicrobial substances like fatty acids and bacteriocins, as well as the generation of cross-reactive antibodies that help prevent infections [18, 19]. In light of all the advantages offered by the normal human microbiota, inappropriate use of antimicrobials can be detrimental to their survival, consequently indirectly impacting the regular functioning of the body, cognitive processes, metabolism, and other bodily functions. Changes in the gut microbiome and the invasion of drug-resistant pathogens can lead to their proliferation, ultimately emerging as the primary internal source of healthcare-associated infections (HAIs) in hospitalized and critically ill patients. Prolonged exposure to specific categories of antibiotics sets the stage for the emergence of *Clostridioides difficile*-associated diarrhea (CDAD) and pseudomembranous colitis. Antibiotics commonly associated with CDAD include fluoroquinolones, cephalosporins, clindamycin, and penicillins. Furthermore, the occurrence of *Clostridioides difficile*-related diarrhea is occasionally linked to extended usage of macrolides, trimethoprim, and sulfonamides and, in rare instances, to the use of aminoglycosides, tetracyclines, chloramphenicol, metronidazole, and vancomycin. Given that a majority of frequently utilized antibiotics can lead to CDAD, a cautious and prudent approach is essential to prevent the rise and dissemination of *Clostridioides difficile* within healthcare settings. It is imperative to implement contact isolation measures, employ targeted antibiotics against C. difficile, and ensure stringent hand hygiene practices to effectively combat stubborn toxigenic strains of *C. difficile* [23, 24]. Notably, *C. difficile* spores exhibit resistance to low- and intermediate-level disinfectants, underscoring the critical need for vigilant monitoring and thorough implementation of cleaning and disinfection protocols. The encounter with ESCAPE pathogens (*Enterococcus faecium*, *Staphylococcus aureus*, *Clostridioides difficile*, *Acinetobacter baumannii*, *Pseudomonas aeruginosa*, and *Enterobacteriaceae*) is a common scenario in healthcare facilities, particularly in intensive care units (ICUs), owing to prolonged exposure to antibiotics, colonization with multidrug-resistant (MDR) pathogens, and preexisting comorbidities. Once these pathogens establish themselves in ICUs, eliminating them from the environment becomes exceedingly challenging. Their ability to thrive in environmental niches, coupled with poor adherence to hand hygiene practices and various other lapses in infection control measures, facilitates the rapid transmission of ESCAPE pathogens within ICUs. These challenges have led to the emergence of extensively drug-resistant gram-negative bacteria and multidrug-resistant *Candida auris* in recent times [25, 26].

8.4 Need for AMSP in Critical Care Units

The prominence of the antimicrobial stewardship program (AMSP) in India was brought to light following the renowned "Chennai Declaration" of 2012 by Ghafur et al., which was succeeded by the implementation of a 5-year plan in 2015. Prior to this, the general populace in India had very little awareness regarding the significant burden of antimicrobial resistance (AMR), and it was not considered a priority issue. The core essence of the 2015 "Chennai Declaration" was centered around the formulation of a comprehensive set of 1-, 2-, and 5-year strategies aimed at addressing the issue of AMR in India. This strategic plan was designed with specific timelines to achieve targeted goals at a national level, involving a wide array of stakeholders, collaborators, organizations, and other entities. At an institutional level, the implementation of AMSP necessitates a collaborative effort among infectious disease specialists, physicians, surgeons, pharmacists, and microbiologists.

The urgency for the implementation of AMSP stemmed from the alarming statistic that 30–60% of antibiotics are often misused or improperly administered, either in terms of dosage, timing, or appropriateness of indication. While these data primarily reflect practices in Western countries, it is reasonable to infer that the rates could be even higher in the context of India. One of the primary objectives of AMSP is to ensure the judicious and appropriate use of antibiotics. The concept of the "30% rule," introduced as early as 2007, highlighted that approximately 30% of hospitalized patients are prescribed antibiotics at any given time, and around 30% of pharmacy expenses are attributed to antibiotic procurement. These percentages are notably higher in the Indian setting, contributing to adverse patient outcomes and increased healthcare costs.

Conversely, the effective implementation of AMSP has the potential to lead to substantial cost savings, with estimates suggesting that pharmacy expenses could be reduced by 10–30% by adhering to the principles of antimicrobial stewardship. In the Indian context, Schedule H drugs have been identified and cataloged, comprising a list of antibiotics that fall under this regulated category. These medications are restricted from being sold without a valid prescription from a healthcare provider. Furthermore, a significant governmental initiative involved the prohibition of unauthorized combinations of antibiotics produced and marketed by pharmaceutical companies, as these combinations tend to exacerbate the issue of AMR rather than mitigate it. Despite the evident benefits and positive impacts of AMSP, it is crucial to delve into the practical challenges and obstacles, particularly in critical care settings, to ensure effective and sustained implementation of antimicrobial stewardship measures.

Antibiotics utilized for empiric therapy in intensive care units are typically broad-spectrum in nature, providing coverage against a wide range of pathogens commonly encountered in such settings. The utilization of these broad-spectrum antibiotics, without appropriate de-escalation strategies, can lead to the emergence of drug-resistant pathogens within the ICU environment. Hence, it is crucial to obtain and analyze suitable samples for culture before initiating antibiotic therapy as this step plays a pivotal role in facilitating the de-escalation process. Subsequently, once susceptibility reports are obtained, it is imperative to de-escalate the empirically prescribed broad-spectrum antibiotics. In cases where there is no indication of microbial growth or infection, it is recommended to discontinue the antibiotic treatment promptly. The unwarranted administration of broad-spectrum antibiotics can disrupt the normal flora of the intestines and promote the proliferation of resistant organisms in the gastrointestinal tract, a phenomenon known as selective antibiotic pressure. Consequently, patients who become colonized with these drug-resistant pathogens are at a higher risk of developing infections caused by multidrug-resistant organisms. To mitigate the risk of fostering drug-resistant pathogens, it is essential to discontinue antibiotics when there are no clinical signs of infection. The excessive use of antibiotics can inflict more harm than benefit on patients. The role of critical care consultants as antimicrobial stewards becomes particularly significant in situations where unnecessary antibiotic therapy needs to be discontinued or de-escalated.

In order to assist healthcare providers in selecting the most appropriate antibiotics in a timely manner, it is advisable to adhere to national antibiotic prescribing guidelines. Critical care consultants and other healthcare practitioners should stay informed about the latest updates in these guidelines, which are continuously revised based on emerging patterns of antimicrobial resistance. National guidelines are designed to be user-friendly and are more pertinent to the Indian healthcare landscape as compared to guidelines formulated in Western countries, which may not fully address the unique antimicrobial resistance challenges prevalent in India. Additionally, it is essential to recognize that India is a significant hub for antimicrobial resistance, with higher rates of resistance observed in comparison to Western nations. Furthermore, healthcare professionals should familiarize themselves with the antibiotic policies established by their respective healthcare facilities and diligently adhere to these protocols with guidance from infectious disease specialists or clinical microbiologists. Active engagement through interactions, case deliberations, and interdisciplinary meetings is imperative to promote the prudent utilization of antibiotics and enhance clinicians' understanding of any emerging patterns of resistance within their healthcare units.

8.5 Drug Discovery Pipeline

Whenever a novel antibiotic is developed, the primary focus lies in targeting critical priority pathogens, which are essential due to the scarcity of effective antibiotics to combat infections caused by these microbes owing to their high resistance rates. The terms multidrug-resistant (MDR), extensively drug-resistant (XDR), and pan-drug-resistant (PDR) play a significant role in characterizing these critical priority pathogens. MDR refers to resistance against three or more classes of antimicrobials, while XDR signifies resistance against most tested antimicrobial classes, and PDR indicates resistance against all antimicrobial agents. According to the 2017 WHO report, the top three critical priority bugs are carbapenem-resistant *Acinetobacter baumannii*, carbapenem-resistant *Pseudomonas aeruginosa*, and carbapenem-resistant/third-generation cephalosporin-resistant (ESBL) *Enterobacteriaceae*.

The availability and cost of these new antibiotics in India raise concerns regarding their utility. The major hindrances associated with any newly approved antimicrobial agent are primarily related to cost and accessibility. Despite the potential effectiveness of these agents against critical priority pathogens commonly encountered in critical care settings, their ability to combat resistance in the long term remains uncertain and requires vigilant observation. The depletion of the existing antibiotic reserve due to misuse and overuse emphasizes the necessity of exercising caution in the utilization of newer antimicrobial agents, ideally limiting their prescription to clinicians with specialized expertise.

8.6 Role of POCTS in Antimicrobial Stewardship Program

Diagnostic stewardship, as the foundation of antibiotic reporting, plays a crucial role in influencing various aspects of antibiotic prescription, such as escalation and de-escalation. The key elements of diagnostic stewardship encompass several important practices. Firstly, it involves the collection of culture specimens before starting antibiotic treatment. Secondly, it emphasizes the appropriate selection of diagnostic tests for timely and accurate diagnosis. Thirdly, it stresses the importance of avoiding unnecessary sampling of cultures. Additionally, diagnostic stewardship includes the critical analysis of culture reports to determine the necessity of initiating antibiotics and the utilization of biomarkers to support judicious antibiotic use. The integration of diagnostic stewardship with antimicrobial stewardship is essential for optimizing the use of antibiotics in clinical settings.

8.7 Procalcitonin (PCT)

Given the limited availability of point-of-care tests for infectious syndromes, the utilization of these tests relies heavily on the clinical judgment of healthcare providers. Various common and emerging point-of-care devices are currently being used in clinical practice. For instance, one notable point-of-care test is procalcitonin (PCT), a precursor of calcitonin that shows increased levels in response to bacterial infections. PCT levels typically begin to rise within 4 h after infection onset and peak between 8 and 24 h later. A normal PCT value of 2 ng/mL suggests a high risk of systemic infection and the potential progression to sepsis. Conversely, a PCT value exceeding 10 ng/mL indicates severe sepsis and septic shock. It is important to note that procalcitonin is more indicative of gram-negative infections. Moreover, procalcitonin serves a valuable function in monitoring treatment progress and serves as a useful indicator for de-escalating antibiotic therapy when appropriate.

8.8 Lactate

Lactate, the final product of anaerobic metabolism, is indicative of tissue hypoxia or shock when present in the body. Levels of serum lactate that measure below 1 mg/dL are generally considered to be within the normal range, while higher concentrations are associated with a less favorable prognosis. In cases of sepsis, lactate serves as a crucial marker for predicting patient outcomes. Utilizing lactate levels as an indicator allows healthcare providers to assess the severity of the condition and make informed decisions regarding treatment strategies.

8.9 Interleukin 6

Interleukin 6 (IL6), classified as a proinflammatory cytokine, is one of the earliest measurable indicators of sepsis, showing an increase within a mere 2 h of onset. This rapid elevation of IL6 makes it a valuable tool in the timely initiation of empiric antibiotic therapy for individuals suspected of having sepsis. Furthermore, interleukin 6 plays a role in stimulating the production of C-reactive protein by the liver. By combining IL6 with other diagnostic markers, healthcare professionals can effectively differentiate between bacterial infections and other inflammatory disorders, leading to more accurate and targeted treatment approaches.

Upon ruling out noninfectious causes, the appropriate use of antibiotics can be ensured, reducing the risk of unnecessary antibiotic use. This approach also helps in preventing the overuse of broad-spectrum antimicrobials, which have been linked to the development of drug-resistant bacterial strains in the gastrointestinal tract. IL6 not only aids in the diagnosis of sepsis but also proves to be valuable in monitoring the progression of the condition and adjusting antibiotic regimens accordingly. Its multifaceted role in patient care highlights the significance of IL6 as a versatile marker in the realm of infectious diseases.

8.10 Summary: The Way Forward

Certain guidelines need to be adhered to for the implementation and application of antimicrobial stewardship programs (AMSP) in critical care settings. One of the key steps is to refrain from the use of high-end antibiotics and instead opt for appropriate empiric antibiotics based on established guidelines. It is advisable to seek recommendations from an expert panel comprising consultants, infectious disease (ID) physicians, and clinical microbiologists before resorting to high-end antibiotics. Another important practice is antibiotic cycling, which plays a significant role in preserving the efficacy of commonly used antibiotics by alleviating the antibiotic pressure resulting from their excessive use. In order to facilitate the prescription of antibiotics in ICUs, it is essential to obtain a specialized antibiogram tailored specifically for the ICU setting, possibly categorized by specimen type. Once culture reports become available, it is imperative to de-escalate antibiotics promptly. In cases where the culture report yields negative results, all antibiotic treatments should be discontinued. Employing point-of-care devices judiciously can aid in the de-escalation of antibiotics, contributing to optimal patient care. Laboratories should consider investing in automated systems for identification and susceptibility testing to expedite the turnaround time for results. The early adoption of molecular tests for diagnosis can lead to a reduction in the duration of antibiotic therapy, promoting better patient outcomes. Developing a mobile application for smartphones that contains comprehensive information on antibiotic spectrum, antibiogram data, and hospital antibiotic policies can be beneficial for both junior doctors and consultants in making informed antibiotic decisions. Rigorous infection control measures, such as cohorting patients, implementing barrier nursing techniques, practicing strict hand hygiene, and enforcing contact isolation protocols for multidrug-resistant (MDR) pathogens, are crucial for preventing cross-transmission of infections within ICUs. Screening patients at high risk and performing colonization screenings before medical procedures for drug-resistant pathogens like methicillin-resistant

Staphylococcus aureus (MRSA) and carbapenem-resistant *Enterobacteriaceae* (CRE) can help in predicting infections in colonized patients. Encouraging and empowering nurses and other allied health staff in ICUs to act as stewards for monitoring infection control practices and promoting compliance with hand hygiene protocols is pivotal. Lastly, continuous training and educational programs focused on reinforcing infection control practices are essential to effectively curb the spread of multidrug-resistant organisms.

8.11 Conclusion

Antibiotics, often referred to as miraculous remedies, wield immense power in combating various infections but can unleash catastrophic consequences if administered inappropriately. The concept of antimicrobial stewardship underscores the crucial role that each individual play in ensuring the judicious use of these potent drugs, a skill that can be honed to perfection through consistent application in daily clinical practice. The implementation of an antimicrobial stewardship program yields a substantial impact on patient outcomes, mortality rates associated with healthcare-associated infections (HAIs), hospital financial performance, national economy, workforce productivity, and other vital aspects of the healthcare system. The escalating threat of antimicrobial resistance has already claimed the well-being of countless individuals, amplifying concerns about the future landscape of healthcare by drastically narrowing down the pool of effective antibiotics available for treatment. Safeguarding this dwindling reservoir of antibiotics emerges as a formidable challenge that demands immediate attention and strategic interventions. The introduction of novel antibiotics into clinical practice necessitates strict adherence to established guidelines and a cautious, prudent approach to their utilization to mitigate the risks of further exacerbating antimicrobial resistance trends.

References

1. Antimicrobial Stewardship Program guideline. Indian Council of Medical Research; 2018. p. 1–62.
2. Walia K, Ohri VC, Mathai D. Antimicrobial Stewardship Programme (AMSP) practices in India. Indian J Med Res. 2015;142(2):130–8. https://doi.org/10.4103/0971-5916.164228.
3. Treatment guidelines for antimicrobial use in common syndromes. New Delhi: Indian Council of Medical Research, Department of Health Research; 2017.
4. Woodhead M, Blasi F, Ewig S, Garau J, Huchon G, Ieven M, et al. Guidelines for the management of adult lower respiratory tract infections. Clin Microbiol Infect. 2011;17:E1–59. https://doi.org/10.1111/j.1469-0691.2011.03672.x.
5. Khilnani GC, Zirpe K, Hadda V, Mehta Y, Madan K, Kulkarni A, et al. Guidelines for antibiotic prescription in intensive care unit. Indian J Crit Care Med. 2019;23(Suppl 1):1–63. https://doi.org/10.5005/jp-journals-10071-23101.

6. No time to wait: securing the future from drug-resistant infections. Report to the secretary-general of the united nations; April 2019. https://www.who.int/news-room/detail/29-04-2019-new-report-calls-for-urgent-action-to-avert-antimicrobialresistance-crisis. Accessed 20 May 2019.
7. Jevons MP. "Celbenin"-resistant staphylococci. Br Med J. 1961;1(5219):124.
8. Yue Z, Zhang J, Zhou Z, Ding C, Zhang T, Wan L, Wang X. Antibiotic degradation dominates the removal of antibiotic resistance genes during composting. Bioresour Technol. 2022;344:126229.
9. Gandra S, Mojica N, Klein EY, Ashok A, Nerurkar V, Kumari M, Ramesh U, Dey S, Vadwai V, Das BR, Laxminarayan R. Trends in antibiotic resistance among major bacterial pathogens isolated from blood cultures tested at a large private laboratory network in India, 2008–2014. Int J Infect Dis. 2016;50:75–82.
10. Bhutani N, Muraleedharan C, Talreja D, Rana SW, Walia S, Kumar A, Walia SK. Occurrence of multidrug resistant extended spectrum beta-lactamase-producing bacteria on iceberg lettuce retailed for human consumption. Biomed Res Int. 2015;2015(1):547547.
11. Hiramatsu K, Hanaki H, Ino T, Yabuta K, Oguri T, Tenover FC. Methicillin-resistant Staphylococcus aureus clinical strain with reduced vancomycin susceptibility. J Antimicrob Chemother. 1997;40(1):135–6. https://doi.org/10.1093/jac/40.1.135.
12. Centers for Disease Control and Prevention (CDC). Staphylococcus aureus resistant to vancomycin. United States, 2002. MMWR Morb Mortal Wkly Rep. 2002;51:565–7.
13. Leclercq R, Derlot E, Duval J, Courvalin P. Plasmid-mediated resistance to vancomycin and teicoplanin in enterococcus faecium. N Engl J Med. 1988;319(3):157–61. https://doi.org/10.1056/NEJM198807213190307.
14. Knothe H, Shah P, Krcmery V, Antal M, Mitsuhashi S. Transferable resistance to cefotaxime, cefoxitin, cefamandole and cefuroxime in clinical isolates of Klebsiella pneumoniae and Serratia marcescens. Infection. 1983;11(6):315–7. https://doi.org/10.1007/BF01641355.
15. Garcia MM. Carbapenemases: a real threat. APUA Newslett. 2013;31:4–6.
16. Liu YY, Wang Y, Walsh TR, Yi LX, Zhang R, Spencer J, et al. Emergence of plasmid-mediated colistin resistance mechanism MCR-1 in animals and human beings in China: a microbiological and molecular biological study. Lancet Infect Dis. 2016;16(2):161–8. https://doi.org/10.1016/S1473-3099(15)00424-7.
17. Davey P, Marwick CA, Scott CL, Charani E, McNeil K, Brown E, et al. Interventions to improve antibiotic prescribing practices for hospital inpatients. Cochrane Database Syst Rev. 2017;2:CD003543. https://doi.org/10.1002/14651858.CD003543.pub4.
18. Cho I, Blaser MJ. The human microbiome: at the interface of health and disease. Nat Rev Genet. 2012;13(4):260–70. https://doi.org/10.1038/nrg3182.
19. Grice EA, Segre JA. The human microbiome: our second genome. Annu Rev Genomics Hum Genet. 2012;13(1):151–70. https://doi.org/10.1146/annurev-genom-090711-163814.
20. What is antimicrobial stewardship? Antimicrobial stewardship from principles to practice. Birmingham: British Society for Antimicrobial Chemotherapy; 2018. p. 44.
21. Teng C, Reveles KR, Obodozie-Ofoegbu O, Frei CR. Clostridium difficile infection risk with important antibiotic classes: an analysis of the FDA adverse event reporting system. Int J Med Sci. 2019;16(5):630–5. https://doi.org/10.7150/ijms.30739.
22. Peterson LR. Bad bugs, no drugs: no ESCAPE revisited. Clin Infect Dis. 2009;49(6):992–3. https://doi.org/10.1086/605539.
23. Chennai Declaration Team. "Chennai declaration": 5-year plan to tackle the challenge of anti-microbial resistance. Indian J Med Microbiol. 2014;32(3):221–8. https://doi.org/10.4103/0255-0857.129053.
24. Magill SS, Edwards JR, Beldavs ZG, Dumyati G, Janelle SJ, Kainer MA, et al. Prevalence of antimicrobial use in US acute care hospitals. JAMA. 2014;312(14):1438–46. https://doi.org/10.1001/jama.2014.12923.

25. Practical guide to antimicrobial stewardship in hospitals. http://bsac.org.uk/wp-content/uploads/2013/07/StewardshipBooklet-Practical-Guide-to-Antimicrobial-Stewardship-in-Hospitals. Accessed 27 May 2019.
26. Guidelines for the management of adults with hospital-acquired, ventilator-associated, and healthcare-associated pneumonia. Am J Respir Crit Care Med. 2005;171(4):388–416. https://doi.org/10.1164/rccm.200405.

Chapter 9
Challenges Faced in Prevention and Management of Healthcare-Acquired Pneumonia (HAP) and Ventilator-Associated Pneumonia (VAP)

9.1 Introduction

Ventilator-associated pneumonia (VAP) manifests itself subsequent to a minimum duration of 48 h post the insertion of an endotracheal tube. Predominantly, the causative agents responsible for VAP comprise gram-negative bacilli and *Staphylococcus aureus*, with a notable emphasis on antibiotic-resistant strains that pose a significant therapeutic challenge. In ventilated patients, the onset of pneumonia typically presents with fever, elevation in white blood cell count, deterioration in oxygen saturation levels, and an escalation in the volume of tracheal secretions, often characterized by purulent qualities. The diagnosis of VAP hinges on a clinical suspicion based on the symptomatic profile exhibited by the patient, complemented by findings from chest radiography, and occasionally substantiated by the identification of identical pathogens in both blood cultures and respiratory specimens or through bronchoscopic assessment of the lower respiratory tract involving quantitative gram staining and culture analysis. The cornerstone of management for VAP revolves around the administration of appropriate antibiotics, albeit the overall prognosis tends to be unfavorable, partly attributable to the presence of concomitant medical conditions [1].

Ventilator-associated pneumonia represents a specific subtype of pneumonia that emerges after an interval of at least 48 h following the placement of an endotracheal tube. This distinctive category falls within the broader spectrum of hospital-acquired pneumonia, encompassing instances of pneumonia occurring in hospitalized patients who are not reliant on mechanical ventilation for respiratory support. VAP is frequently characterized by the involvement of more resilient pathogens and a higher incidence of adverse clinical outcomes compared to other variants of hospital-acquired pneumonia.

R. Chakraverty, A. K. Kundu, *Hospital-Acquired Infections in Intensive Care Unit and their Management*, https://doi.org/10.1007/978-981-96-0018-2_9

9.2 Epidemiological Perspectives of Hospital-Acquired Pneumonia

The definitions of hospital-acquired pneumonia (HAP) and ventilator-associated pneumonia (VAP) exhibit variations and lack consistency, which can impact the reported incidences significantly. In the context of this discourse, HAP is defined as occurring after 48 h from hospital admission, either in the intensive care unit (ICU) or hospital ward, regardless of mechanical ventilation (MV) association. The term HAP is specifically used to describe cases unrelated to MV or intubation, distinguishing it from VAP, which manifests after 48 h of MV support. A patient exhibiting symptoms of lower respiratory tract infection after more than 48 h under MV, without chest X-ray opacities, receives a diagnosis of ventilator-associated tracheobronchitis (VAT).

Respiratory infections, particularly HAP and VAP, represent the most common nosocomial infections encountered in ICU settings. A noteworthy global multicenter study revealed that half of the observed patients had an infection, with 65% originating from the respiratory system. In a prevalence study conducted across 183 US hospitals, HAP and VAP accounted for 22% of all hospital infections. Research indicates that 10–40% of patients undergoing MV for over 48 h are at risk of developing VAP, with variations in incidence rates influenced by diagnostic challenges, diverse definitions, diagnostic methodologies, and patient populations (e.g., those with ARDS, brain damage, or undergoing VA-ECMO) [2].

Significant variations in VAP incidence rates have been documented between European and US ICUs. The National Healthcare Safety Network (NHSN) reported VAP rates of 1–2.5 cases per 1000 days of MV in the USA, notably lower than the European rate of 8.9 episodes per 1000 days of MV according to the European Centre for Disease Prevention and Control (ECDC). Spain's ENVIN-HELICS 2018 report noted an incidence of 5.87 episodes per 1000 days of MV. Both regions have seen a gradual decline in VAP incidence, likely attributed to preventive measures, though potential biases due to monitoring criteria subjectivity cannot be dismissed.

Ventilator-associated tracheobronchitis (VAT) is emerging as a condition of increasing importance in clinical settings. A prospective multicenter study revealed similar incidence rates for VAT and VAP, with 10.2 and 8.8 episodes per 1000 days of mechanical ventilation, respectively. Distinguishing between VAT and VAP can pose challenges, with some experts suggesting a continuum between the two conditions and the possibility of VAT progressing to VAP. This hypothesis is supported by several factors, including higher VAP incidence in VAT patients, shared post-mortem findings, elevated biomarker levels and severity scores in VAP cases compared to VAT, as well as similarities in microbiological profiles and mortality rates.

Non-ventilated patients in the ICU demonstrate a reduced likelihood of developing pneumonia, as evidenced by a recent study where it was observed that 40% of pneumonia cases acquired in the ICU were found in patients who had not undergone ventilation previously. This finding sheds light on the potential impact of ventilation on pneumonia development within ICU settings. Another research conducted across

400 German ICUs highlighted a VAP rate of 5.44 per 1000 days of mechanical ventilation (MV), contrasting with lower rates of 1.58 per 1000 days for noninvasive mechanical ventilation (NIMV) and 1.15 per 1000 for hospital-acquired pneumonia (HAP) patients. These statistics underscore the varying risks associated with different ventilation methods in the ICU environment [3, 4].

The global incidence of HAP, encompassing both intra- and extra-ICU cases, presents a wide range of 5 to over 20 cases per 1000 hospital admissions, making it challenging to ascertain due to discrepancies in definitions and methodologies employed. Analysis by the European Centre for Disease Prevention and Control (ECDC) based on data from 947 hospitals in 30 countries revealed a prevalence of HAP at 1.3% (95% CI, 1.2–1.3%). In contrast, a study in the United States documented a HAP frequency of 1.6% among hospitalized patients, with an incidence density of 3.63 per 1000 patient-days, emphasizing regional variations in pneumonia rates within healthcare facilities. Furthermore, a multicenter study in Spain examining 165 cases of extra-ICU HAP reported an incidence rate ranging from 3.1 (1.3–5.9) episodes per 1000 admissions, highlighting the influence of hospital factors and patient characteristics on pneumonia occurrence [5].

Within the subgroup of non-ventilated patients, when microbial cultures are accessible, the etiology of pneumonia mirrors that of VAP, with prevalent pathogens such as *Pseudomonas aeruginosa*, *Staphylococcus aureus*, and various species of *Enterobacteriaceae*. This emphasizes the importance of understanding the microbial landscape in pneumonia cases among non-ventilated ICU patients for effective management strategies. Additionally, the specific microbial composition may vary depending on the severity of the patient's condition, individual risk factors, and the prevailing epidemiological factors in the local healthcare setting. This nuanced understanding of pneumonia etiology underscores the complexity of infection dynamics in critically ill patients and the need for tailored approaches to combat these healthcare-associated infections.

9.3 Patient Outcomes and Impact

According to findings from a case-control study, patients diagnosed with hospital-acquired pneumonia (HAP) exhibited a more severe clinical course compared to non-HAP patients. This included a significantly higher mortality rate of 19% as opposed to 3.9% in non-HAP cases, a greater frequency of ICU admissions at 56.3% vs. 22.8%, and an extended hospital stay of 15.9 days vs. 4.4 days for non-HAP patients. Overall, the odds ratio of mortality for patients with HAP was found to be 8.4 times higher than those without HAP. Historically, it has been commonly believed that mortality rates are higher in ventilator-associated pneumonia (VAP) cases compared to HAP instances. However, when intensive care unit (ICU)-related HAP was contrasted with VAP cases, the raw mortality rates appeared comparable, indicating a stronger association with patient-specific factors rather than prior intubation. Analysis of data from ten recent clinical trials focusing on

ICU patients highlighted higher mortality rates for HAP cases requiring mechanical ventilation, relatively lower rates for VAP cases, and even lesser rates for HAP patients not needing ventilation support. The requirement for intubation in such cases is often considered a significant indicator of unfavorable pneumonia progression [6].

Adjusted mortality rates were found to be alike for VAP and ventilated HAP cases, suggesting similar outcomes in these scenarios. A recent extensive multicenter study encompassing over 14,000 patients sought to explore the impact of VAP and HAP within the ICU setting, revealing that both conditions were linked to an elevated risk of death within 30 days. The hazard ratios for mortality stood at 1.38 (1.24–1.52) for VAP and 1.82 (1.35–2.45) for HAP cases, accentuating the gravity of these infections in critical care. Reports have also indicated a mortality rate of 13% for HAP cases, along with a noticeable increase in hospital stay from 4 to 16 days and a surge in costs by $40,000 per episode. VAP cases have similarly been associated with prolonged stays in the ICU and hospital, alongside extended durations of mechanical ventilation. The mortality rates for VAP patients have shown variability, ranging from 24 to 72%, with notably higher mortality rates seen in cases caused by *Pseudomonas aeruginosa* [7–9].

Newer data has estimated an attributable mortality of 13% in VAP cases, particularly elevated in patients with moderate severity levels and those undergoing surgical procedures. Ventilator-associated tracheobronchitis (VAT) has been correlated in various studies with extended ICU stays and prolonged periods of mechanical ventilation. Nevertheless, the absence of randomized controlled trials demonstrating the efficacy of treatment in VAT cases remains a significant gap in current knowledge. Furthermore, while higher mortality rates have not been consistently observed in patients experiencing this complication, the impact on clinical outcomes necessitates further investigation [10].

9.4 Risk Factors for HAP

Traditionally, three categories of risk factors contributing to nosocomial pneumonia have been traditionally identified: those associated with patients, those related to infection prevention, and those connected to medical procedures. Patient-related risk factors involve various conditions such as severe acute or chronic illnesses, coma, malnutrition, prolonged hospitalization, hypertension, metabolic acidosis, smoking habits, and complications stemming from central nervous system disorders like COPDs, diabetes, alcoholism, chronic kidney failure, and respiratory insufficiency. In terms of risk factors related to infection prevention, shortcomings in hand hygiene practices and improper maintenance of respiratory support equipment are notable. Moreover, factors associated with surgical interventions include the use of sedatives, corticosteroids, and other immunosuppressive agents, as well as prolonged surgical procedures, particularly those involving the chest or abdomen, and prolonged or inappropriate courses of antibiotics. Recent research has highlighted that the risk of nodular pneumonia escalates among patients who receive gastric acid-modifying medications during their hospital stay.

In the absence of artificial airways, pneumonia occurring in patients undergoing noninvasive mechanical ventilation can be classified as a subtype of noncirculating pneumonia. An extensive prospective analysis encompassing 520 individuals undergoing noninvasive mechanical ventilation was conducted. The study findings did not reveal any statistically significant variances in age, gender distribution, disease severity, or gas exchange parameters between patients who developed nosocomial pneumonia or complications related to noninvasive mechanical ventilation and those who did not [11].

9.5 Prognosis and Outcomes [12]

Pneumonia acquired in the intensive care unit (ICU) has a detrimental impact on mortality rates, leading to prolonged hospital stays and increased mechanical ventilation (MV) duration, particularly in cases of ventilator-associated pneumonia (VAP). Consequently, this results in escalated healthcare costs. The correlation between the onset of nosocomial pneumonia and the rise in mortality remains a topic of debate within the medical community. Several factors are linked to a worsened prognosis in pneumonia cases, including the presence of complications, the overall performance of the patient, the severity of infection at the onset, and the patient's response to the infection. However, studies often overlook these factors when analyzing the impact of suitable empirical antibiotic usage. The selection of inappropriate antibiotic therapy is directly associated with the presence of multidrug-resistant organisms (MDRO), which could be a crucial and significant predictor. Inappropriately treated patients with severe infections face significantly higher mortality rates. Therefore, a comprehensive assessment of prognostic factors should prioritize patients who have received suitable empirical treatments. Subsequently, it is essential to consider two potential clinical scenarios to evaluate patient-related factors and disease-related aspects or conduct more dynamic analyses to identify which clinical trajectories are linked to inadequate treatment responses and consequently, poorer outcomes. Factors such as advanced age, underlying hemodynamic malignancies, or clinical presentations like septic shock or acute respiratory failure are correlated with increased mortality rates, yet these associations have limited clinical relevance. Similar patterns are observed in analytical aspects, such as initial lymphopenia.

There is a growing interest in evaluating responses to early treatment interventions. Recently, Esperatti and his colleagues validated the connection between various clinical parameters measured 72–96 h posttreatment initiation and the prognosis of 335 patients with nosocomial pneumonia. Patients with unfavorable clinical outcomes commonly exhibit factors such as lack of improved oxygenation, requirement for mechanical ventilation in hospital-acquired pneumonia (HAP) cases, persistent fever and hypothermia, presence of respiratory secretions, radiological involvement exceeding 50% of lung regions, septic shock, or multi-organ failure post-antibiotic therapy, leading to extended hospital stays, prolonged mechanical ventilation, and increased mortality rates. Among these factors, the absence of improved oxygen levels is significantly linked to higher mortality rates (OR 2.18 [1.24–3.84] $p = 0.007$). Both initial assessments and 72–96 h monitoring using criteria like Clinical Pulmonary Infection Score (CPIS) or biomarkers such as C-reactive proteins or procalcitonin are widely recognized for their prognostic value and infection monitoring purposes.

9.6 MDR Pathogen and Colonization

MDR *Pseudomonas aeruginosa*, enterobacteria producing beta-lactamase (ESBL-E), enterobacteria producing *Staphylococcus aureus* (MRSA), *Acinetobacter baumannii*, and enterobacteria producing carbapenemase (CPE) are the multidrug resistant organisms (MDROs) that play a significant role in hospital-acquired pneumonia (HAP). It is crucial to have a thorough understanding of the local epidemiology due to substantial variations in the prevalence of each MDRO within different regions. The ENVIN-HELICS report provides a quantitative assessment of the resistance patterns exhibited by the most critical microorganisms against various antibiotics, offering a comprehensive overview of the anticipated resistance rates for nosocomial pneumonia specifically in the Spanish intensive care units (ICUs) [13].

The data derived from ENVIN-HELICS also reveals a remarkable surge in the resistance of *Klebsiella* bacteria to carbapenems, signifying a concerning trend in recent years. Conversely, there has been a consistent resistance level to antibiotics noted in the remaining bacterial strains. When evaluating the risk factors associated with the development of nosocomial pneumonia attributed to MDROs within the ICU, it is essential to conduct an initial analysis of the factors linked to these pathogens. The guidelines established by European regulatory bodies concerning nosocomial pneumonia encompass risk elements associated with MDROs, including septic shock, high prevalence of MDROs in healthcare facilities, prior antibiotic exposure, prolonged hospital stays (over 5 days), and previous colonization by MDROs. These risk factors are broadly applicable across various MDRO types; however, to distinguish between different strains of MDROs, particular emphasis is placed on local epidemiological data and the patient's history of MDRO colonization. The significance of colonization as a risk factor for acquiring pneumonia caused by the colonizing microorganism varies depending on the specific MDRO type and the site of colonization.

9.7 Etiology

The predominant etiology of ventilator-associated pneumonia (VAP) can be attributed to the phenomenon of microaspiration, whereby bacteria residing in the oropharynx and upper respiratory tract of critically ill individuals are inadvertently inhaled into the lower airways due to compromised respiratory defenses and the use of mechanical ventilation. This process of bacterial colonization and subsequent aspiration poses a significant risk for the development of pneumonia in patients requiring intensive care interventions.

9.8 Risk Factors

Endotracheal intubation represents a significant risk factor when it comes to the development of ventilator-associated pneumonia. This invasive procedure disrupts the natural defenses of the airway, leading to a compromised ability to cough effectively and impairing the process of mucociliary clearance. Moreover, the presence of an endotracheal tube creates a conducive environment for the microaspiration of secretions containing harmful bacteria, which tend to accumulate above the inflated cuff of the tube. Not only that, but these bacteria have the ability to form biofilms both on and inside the tube itself, providing them with protection against antibiotics and the immune system of the host. The period with the highest susceptibility to VAP spans the initial 10 days following the intubation procedure. It is estimated that ventilator-associated pneumonia affects a considerable proportion of mechanically ventilated patients, with rates ranging from 9% to as high as 27%.

9.9 Pathogens

Pathogens and antibiotic resistance patterns display significant variabilities among different healthcare institutions and even within the same institutions over relatively short periods, such as transitioning from 1 month to the next. It is absolutely essential to have local antibiograms at the institutional level that are consistently and regularly updated to precisely determine the most appropriate empiric antibiotic therapy for patients. The importance of these antibiograms cannot be emphasized enough, as they serve a pivotal role in directing healthcare professionals toward making well-informed decisions regarding antibiotic prescriptions, thereby contributing to the overall quality of patient care.

The identification of predominant pathogens in a specific healthcare environment is foundational for the implementation of effective infection control measures and the provision of optimal patient care. Noteworthy pathogens that deserve attention include enteric gram-negative bacteria, with a particular focus on species like *Enterobacter*, *Klebsiella pneumoniae*, *Escherichia coli*, *Serratia marcescens*, *Proteus* species, and *Acinetobacter* species. These pathogens must be carefully considered due to their potential impact on healthcare settings and patient outcomes, underscoring the necessity for vigilance in their management and treatment.

In instances where pneumonia emerges within a period of 4–7 days following hospital admission, methicillin-sensitive *Staphylococcus aureus*, *Streptococcus pneumoniae*, and *Haemophilus influenzae* stand out as the primary causative agents. Nonetheless, with prolonged intubation or hospitalization, *Pseudomonas aeruginosa*, methicillin-resistant *S. aureus*, and enteric gram-negative organisms become increasingly prevalent. Understanding these evolving trends is critical for devising effective management and treatment strategies within healthcare facilities to address the changing landscape of infectious pathogens.

The ability to recognize the alterations in common pathogens based on the timing of pneumonia onset or the duration of hospital stay is of utmost importance for healthcare providers. By remaining abreast of these shifting patterns, appropriate interventions can be implemented to prevent and manage infections efficiently, ultimately leading to enhanced patient outcomes and reduced morbidity and mortality rates. A history of intravenous antibiotic therapy within the preceding 90 days substantially heightens the probability of encountering antibiotic-resistant organisms, particularly methicillin-resistant *Staphylococcus aureus* and *Pseudomonas aeruginosa* infections in cases of ventilator-associated pneumonia (VAP). This underscores the critical nature of considering prior antibiotic exposure when evaluating and treating patients with suspected VAP, as it can significantly impact the choice and effectiveness of antimicrobial agents employed in such scenarios.

Infection with a resilient microorganism markedly escalates both mortality and morbidity rates among individuals, especially those in critical care settings. Various risk factors contribute to the development of antibiotic-resistant organisms specifically in ventilator-associated pneumonia (VAP), including septic shock occurring at the onset of VAP, acute respiratory distress syndrome (ARDS) manifesting before VAP, hospitalization lasting 5 days or more preceding VAP incidence, and undergoing acute renal replacement therapy before VAP onset. Additionally, the utilization of high-dose corticosteroids heightens the susceptibility to contracting *Legionella* and *Pseudomonas* infections, further complicating the clinical course of patients with VAP. Individuals with chronic suppurative lung conditions such as cystic fibrosis and bronchiectasis face an increased risk of infection by gram-negative pathogens, some of which may exhibit resistance to commonly used antibiotics.

The root cause of pneumonia in critically ill patients undergoing mechanical ventilation typically presents with symptoms such as fever, elevated respiratory rate, changes in heart rate, or alterations in respiratory parameters, like an escalation in purulent secretions or deteriorating hypoxemia. These clinical manifestations serve as crucial indicators for diagnosing pneumonia in this vulnerable patient population, necessitating a thorough evaluation of risk factors and symptoms to guide appropriate management strategies. Particularly in critical care settings, where prompt and accurate diagnosis is paramount for optimizing patient outcomes, healthcare providers must be vigilant in recognizing and addressing these signs of respiratory infections. Understanding the etiology and risk factors associated with antibiotic-resistant organisms in VAP is essential for guiding healthcare professionals in implementing effective preventive measures and selecting the most appropriate treatment strategies to combat these challenging infections. This comprehensive knowledge underscores the significance of a multidisciplinary approach in managing VAP cases, encompassing infection control practices, antimicrobial stewardship initiatives, and individualized treatment regimens tailored to microbial susceptibility profiles. By navigating the intricate interplay between patient characteristics, microbial pathogens, and treatment modalities, healthcare teams can work toward enhancing clinical outcomes and mitigating the impact of antibiotic resistance in critical care environments.

9.10 Diagnosis

- Chest X-ray and clinical criteria (limited accuracy)
- Sometimes bronchoscopy or blood cultures

9.11 Symptoms and Signs

Diagnosis in the medical field is inherently flawed and imperfect, often presenting challenges in accurately pinpointing specific conditions. In clinical settings, the suspicion of ventilator-associated pneumonia (VAP) commonly arises when a new infiltrate is observed on a chest X-ray taken to assess emerging symptoms or signs, such as fever, increased secretions, or deteriorating hypoxemia, or when leukocytosis is detected. Nevertheless, it is crucial to note that no single symptom, sign, or radiographic finding can be deemed entirely sensitive or specific for the diagnosis of VAP, as these manifestations can also be attributed to alternative conditions like atelectasis, pulmonary embolism, or pulmonary edema, all of which may overlap with the clinical presentation of acute respiratory distress syndrome.

Although gram stain and semiquantitative cultures of endotracheal aspirates are not definitive tools for definitively confirming infection, they are recommended for providing valuable guidance in the treatment of VAP. In contrast, bronchoscopic sampling of lower airway secretions for quantitative culture stands out as a more reliable method for procuring specimens that can effectively discriminate between colonization and genuine infection. The insights obtained through bronchoscopic sampling play a crucial role in reducing unnecessary antibiotic usage and facilitating the transition from broader to more targeted antibiotic coverage. However, it is essential to acknowledge that despite these advantages, the use of bronchoscopic sampling has not demonstrated a significant impact on patient outcomes. The assessment of inflammatory mediators in bronchoalveolar lavage fluid or serum has not exhibited consistent reliability in informing decisions regarding the initiation of antibiotic therapy. The sole finding that possesses a high degree of reliability in identifying both pneumonia and the causative pathogen is a positive pleural fluid culture, which is typically obtained through thoracentesis in individuals with pleural effusion. Furthermore, while blood cultures can offer relatively high specificity when a respiratory pathogen is detected, their sensitivity remains limited in certain scenarios.

9.12 Prognosis

The mortality rate associated with ventilator-associated pneumonia remains alarmingly high, despite the presence of highly potent antibiotics that are deemed effective in treating this respiratory infection. Nevertheless, it is crucial to note that not all cases of mortality can be solely attributed to the pneumonia infection; a significant number of fatalities are intricately linked to the patient's pre-existing underlying medical conditions. Research findings have consistently shown that the prompt and appropriate administration of the initial antimicrobial therapy significantly enhances the patient's chances of recovery and survival, thereby underscoring the pivotal role of timely intervention in improving prognosis outcomes. Moreover, the prognosis of individuals suffering from ventilator-associated pneumonia is further compounded in cases where the infection is caused by antibiotic-resistant strains of bacteria, as these microbial pathogens pose a formidable challenge to treatment options, leading to heightened risks of adverse outcomes and increased mortality rates. The emergence of antibiotic resistance in pneumonia-causing bacteria has emerged as a pressing concern in the realm of healthcare, necessitating the development of novel therapeutic strategies and heightened surveillance measures to curb the spread of these resistant strains and mitigate the associated risks of treatment failure and poor prognosis. In light of these complexities, there is an urgent need for a comprehensive and multifaceted approach that encompasses not only the judicious use of antibiotics but also the implementation of stringent infection control measures and the exploration of alternative treatment modalities to effectively combat ventilator-associated pneumonia and its grave implications on patient outcomes.

9.13 Treatment of VAP

In scenarios where there is a suspicion of ventilator-associated pneumonia, the strategy involves the administration of antibiotics chosen through empirical evidence, taking into account factors like local sensitivity patterns and patient-specific risk elements for antibiotic-resistant microorganisms. The guidelines established by the Infectious Diseases Society of America and the American Thoracic Society in 2007 utilized comprehensive criteria to identify the population prone to infection by antibiotic-resistant pathogens. This approach resulted in a significant number of VAP patients needing broad-spectrum antibiotics that target MRSA and resistant *Pseudomonas* strains. However, the most recent guidelines from 2016 emphasize the significance of selecting a more focused range of empiric antibiotics whenever possible. In cases where treatment for VAP is necessary and there are no evident risk factors for antibiotic-resistant organisms, coupled with a low mortality risk, the empiric therapy in a healthcare facility with MRSA incidence below 10–20% and *Pseudomonas aeruginosa* resistance rate lower than 10% for commonly used antipseudomonal antibiotics may include medications like piperacillin/tazobactam, cefepime, levofloxacin, imipenem, or meropenem.

Nevertheless, in healthcare settings where MRSA prevalence exceeds 10–20%, it is recommended to add vancomycin or linezolid to the treatment regimen. For patients with a high mortality risk, those with risk factors for antibiotic-resistant organisms, or in situations where reliable local antibiograms are unavailable, the guidelines propose triple therapy involving two medications effective against *Pseudomonas* and one against MRSA. This could entail an antipseudomonal cephalosporin (cefepime or ceftazidime) or an antipseudomonal carbapenem (imipenem, meropenem) or a beta-lactam/beta-lactamase inhibitor (piperacillin/tazobactam), an antipseudomonal fluoroquinolone (ciprofloxacin or levofloxacin) or an aminoglycoside (amikacin, gentamicin, tobramycin), and linezolid or vancomycin. The inappropriate use of antibiotics significantly contributes to the emergence of antimicrobial resistance; however, the adequacy of initial empiric antibiotic selection plays a crucial role in determining the patient's outcome. Therefore, the treatment strategy should begin with the use of broad-spectrum antibiotics initially, followed by a transition to the most targeted regimen possible based on the patient's clinical response and the findings from cultures and antibiotic susceptibility tests.

9.14 Prevention

There exist several strategies that can be implemented to prevent the occurrence of ventilator-associated pneumonia. One effective measure is the utilization of semi-upright or upright positioning, which has been demonstrated to lower the risk of aspiration and pneumonia when compared to recumbent positioning. This method is considered the simplest and most efficient way to prevent ventilator-associated pneumonia. Another preventive approach involves the application of noninvasive ventilation techniques such as continuous positive airway pressure (CPAP) or bilevel positive airway pressure (BPAP). These methods help in averting the breach in the airway defense that can arise from endotracheal intubation, thereby eliminating the necessity for intubation in certain patients. Moreover, noninvasive ventilation has been linked to a decrease in the incidence of ventilator-associated pneumonia. The continuous removal of subglottic secretions via a specially designed endotracheal tube connected to a suction device is another strategy that can aid in reducing the risk of micro aspiration and the occurrence of VAP. Despite this benefit, it is crucial to note that this intervention does not significantly alter overall clinical outcomes. Similarly, the use of silver-coated endotracheal tubes has been found to diminish biofilm formation and lower the incidence of VAP. Nevertheless, like subglottic secretion removal, the implementation of silver-coated tubes does not bring about substantial changes in overall clinical outcomes.

The controversial practice of selective decontamination of the oropharynx or the entire gastrointestinal tract involves the application of specific agents, such as topical gentamicin, colistin, chlorhexidine, vancomycin cream, polymyxin, aminoglycosides, quinolones, nystatin, or amphotericin B. Despite the potential benefits of reducing VAP incidence, concerns regarding the emergence of resistant strains have hindered widespread acceptance of these decontamination methods. Additionally, there is a lack of conclusive evidence demonstrating a reduction in mortality rates following decontamination practices. Surveillance cultures and the routine replacement of ventilator circuits or endotracheal tubes have not exhibited a significant impact on decreasing the occurrence of ventilator-associated pneumonia. These measures, although commonly implemented in clinical settings, have not been proven to effectively reduce the incidence of VAP.

9.15 Summary

Ventilator-associated pneumonia (VAP) is a type of pneumonia that occurs after a minimum of 48 h following the insertion of an endotracheal tube into the patient. The microorganisms responsible for VAP differ from those typically associated with pneumonia acquired outside of healthcare settings and often necessitate the administration of initial empiric antibiotic treatment that is effective against bacteria resistant to antibiotics. Identifying VAP can be challenging, with the isolation of a potential pathogen from pleural fluid or blood cultures representing the most definitive diagnostic clue. It is recommended to reassess patients within a timeframe of 2–3 days post the commencement of treatment and to consider modifying the antibiotic regimen based on the results of culture tests and clinical evaluations.

References

1. Bassetti M, Righi E, Vena A, Graziano E, Russo A, Peghin M. Risk stratification and treatment of ICU-acquired pneumonia caused by multidrug-resistant/extensively drug-resistant/pandrug-resistant bacteria. Curr Opin Crit Care. 2018;24(5):385–93.
2. Rodríguez-Baño J, Paño-Pardo JR, Alvarez-Rocha L, Asensio A, Calbo E, Cercenado E, et al. Programs for optimizing the use of antibiotics (PROA) in Spanish hospitals: GEIH-SEIMC, SEFH and SEMPSPH consensus document. Enferm Infecc Microbiol Clin. 2012;30(1):22.e1–e23.
3. Tabah A, Cotta MO, Garnacho-Montero J, Schouten J, Roberts JA, Lipman J, et al. A systematic review of the definitions, determinants, and clinical outcomes of antimicrobial de-escalation in the intensive care unit. Clin Infect Dis. 2016;62(8):1009–17.
4. Martin-Loeches I, Povoa P, Nseir S. A way towards ventilator-associated lower respiratory tract infection research. Intensive Care Med. 2020;46:1504. https://doi.org/10.1007/s00134-020-06101-7.
5. Fernando SM, Tran A, Cheng W, Klompas M, Kyeremanteng K, Mehta S, et al. Diagnosis of ventilator-associated pneumonia in critically ill adult patients—a systematic review and meta-analysis. Intensive Care Med. 2020;46:1170. https://doi.org/10.1007/s00134-020-06036-z.
6. Vincent J-L, Rello J, Marshall J, Silva E, Anzueto A, Martin CD, et al. International study of the prevalence and outcomes of infection in intensive care units. JAMA. 2009;302(21):2323–9.

7. Magill SS, Edwards JR, Fridkin SK. Emerging infections program healthcare-associated infections and antimicrobial use prevalence survey team. Survey of health care-associated infections. N Engl J Med. 2014;370(26):2542–3.
8. American Thoracic Society, Infectious Diseases Society of America. Guidelines for the management of adults with hospital-acquired, ventilator-associated, and healthcare-associated pneumonia. Am J Respir Crit Care Med. 2005;171(4):388–416.
9. Forel J-M, Voillet F, Pulina D, Gacouin A, Perrin G, Barrau K, et al. Ventilator-associated pneumonia and ICU mortality in severe ARDS patients ventilated according to a lung-protective strategy. Crit Care. 2012;16(2):R65.
10. Ruiz J, Ramirez P, Gordon M, Villarreal E, Frasquet J, Poveda-Andres JL, et al. Antimicrobial stewardship programme in critical care medicine: a prospective interventional study. Med Int. 2018;42(5):266–73.
11. Asehnoune K, Seguin P, Allary J, Feuillet F, Lasocki S, Cook F, et al. Hydrocortisone and fludrocortisone for prevention of hospital-acquired pneumonia in patients with severe traumatic brain injury (Corti-TC): a double-blind, multicentre phase 3, randomised placebo-controlled trial. Lancet Respir Med. 2014;2(9):706–16.
12. Bouglé A, Bombled C, Margetis D, Lebreton G, Vidal C, Coroir M, et al. Ventilator-associated pneumonia in patients assisted by veno-arterial extracorporeal membrane oxygenation support: epidemiology and risk factors of treatment failure. PLoS One. 2018;13(4):e0194976.
13. Dudeck MA, Weiner LM, Allen-Bridson K, Malpiedi PJ, Peterson KD, Pollock DA, et al. National Healthcare Safety Network (NHSN) report, data summary for 2012, device-associated module. Am J Infect Control. 2013;41(12):1148–6.

Chapter 10
Hospital Infection Control: Work in Progress?

10.1 Introduction

Nosocomial infections and their management present a substantial worldwide challenge that goes beyond mere geographical boundaries. Not only do these infections lead to higher rates of sickness and mortality among patients, but they also result in increased healthcare costs due to the need for more antimicrobial treatments and extended hospital stays. This issue is particularly severe in developing countries with limited resources, where the prevalence of nosocomial infections exceeds 40% [1], further worsening the socioeconomic strain within these regions. The lack of proper infection control measures exacerbates the aforementioned difficulties, creating a harmful cycle of declining healthcare systems. Despite the fact that problematic pathogens like methicillin-resistant *Staphylococcus aureus* (MRSA) and multidrug-resistant (MDR) *Acinetobacter,* as well as nosocomial infections such as bloodstream infections (BSI) and ventilator-associated pneumonia (VAP), are widespread across all nations regardless of their resource availability, the severity of MDR pathogen prevalence and the frequency of nosocomial infections differ significantly due to inadequate infection control protocols. This highlights the crucial necessity of implementing efficient infection control strategies to alleviate the impact of nosocomial infections on both patients and healthcare systems globally [2–4].

10.2 Infection Control

Nosocomial infections present a significant obstacle in the domain of healthcare in Turkey, especially within university hospitals, where the incidence of healthcare-associated infections has been documented at 13.4%, as indicated by recent research [3], and a strikingly high 48.7% within intensive care units [4]. In contrast, the

R. Chakraverty, A. K. Kundu, *Hospital-Acquired Infections in Intensive Care Unit and their Management*, https://doi.org/10.1007/978-981-96-0018-2_10

Netherlands reports a lower prevalence of nosocomial infections at 7.2%, with rates fluctuating between 6.7% and 9.0% in nonacademic and academic settings [5], based on data obtained from the national surveillance system PREZIES. The difference in infection rates observed between the two nations can be linked to the differing infrastructural capacities of their respective healthcare institutions. Turkish medical facilities often face challenges due to insufficient resources, such as a deficiency in single rooms and dedicated isolation units. This lack of proper infrastructure not only hinders the implementation of infection control measures but also fosters the propagation and dissemination of multidrug-resistant pathogens. Furthermore, the absence of controls for temperature, humidity, and air quality further compounds the issue of infection transmission within these healthcare settings.

10.3 A Case Study

The inadequate conditions present in Turkish hospitals are further exacerbated by uncomfortable working environments, especially noticeable during the scorching summer months, which can significantly hinder the effectiveness of healthcare professionals. Moreover, the overcrowding and limited bed-to-bed spacing in hospital wards, especially in critical care units, pose significant obstacles to providing optimal patient care. In the Netherlands, intensive care units maintain a bed-to-bed separation of at least 150 cm; however, Turkish hospitals often fall short with only 100 cm of distance between beds. The congested settings and the constant rotation of patients in Turkish healthcare facilities create barriers to implementing efficient infection control protocols, leading to the continuous spread of multidrug-resistant microorganisms and an increased incidence of healthcare-associated infections. The deficiencies in infrastructure and the overcrowded state of Turkish hospitals highlight the urgent necessity for improved resources and enhanced infection control strategies to reduce the prevalence of nosocomial infections in the nation.

Hand hygiene is considered one of the most critical measures in the control of infections, playing a vital role in the prevention of disease transmission. The adherence to hand hygiene protocols among healthcare workers in Turkey is generally reported to be quite low, with compliance rates falling below 33% [6–8]. This low compliance can be attributed to various factors such as heavy workloads, inadequate facilities like a shortage of sinks, limited access to hygiene products, and behavioral considerations. The challenging situation is further compounded by overcrowding in healthcare facilities and the inadequate number of healthcare workers available to effectively manage the workload. In contrast, the nurse-to-patient ratio in intensive care units in the Netherlands averages 1 to 1, whereas in Turkey, this ratio typically ranges between 1–3 and 1–5. Despite the recognized benefits of using alcoholic hand-rubs for hand disinfection, healthcare workers in Turkey still favor hand washing, which is less time-efficient [9]. The relatively high cost of branded hand-rubs presents a barrier for countries with limited resources, making them less accessible to healthcare facilities. Strategies aimed at enhancing hand hygiene compliance in healthcare settings encompass educational initiatives, the display of hand hygiene promotion posters, and the provision of alcoholic hand-rubs and paper towels. The healthcare infrastructure in the Netherlands, which includes an adequate number of sinks and bedside hand-rub dispensers in ICUs, theoretically allows for complete hand hygiene compliance. Nevertheless, recent studies have revealed that the actual hand hygiene compliance rates [10] in the Netherlands are surprisingly lower than anticipated, averaging only 19%, even falling below the rates observed in Turkey. Factors such as awareness of infection control issues, levels of knowledge, and individual behaviors all contribute significantly to the prevention of healthcare-associated infections [11]. A comparative study on hand hygiene practices during catheter care in ICUs in the Netherlands and Turkey unveiled substantial differences in compliance rates, with Turkey recording an 18% compliance rate compared to 65% in the Netherlands. Despite an educational intervention, there was no notable improvement in hand hygiene compliance in Turkish ICUs, while Dutch facilities witnessed a noticeable increase. However, a recent study conducted in Turkey showcased the effectiveness of regular training for residents responsible for inserting intravascular catheters, as well as nurses and interns involved in catheter maintenance, in reducing the incidence of catheter-related infections in major teaching hospitals. Numerous factors influence human behavior, encompassing family culture, levels of knowledge, beliefs, personality traits, role models, and potential rewards. In countries with limited resources, healthcare workers may lose motivation in their duties due to inadequate financial incentives, resulting in a tendency to adhere strictly to minimum routine tasks. Given that many behavioral patterns are established during childhood, it is crucial to implement hand hygiene promotion programs within the community to educate and instill good practices in future healthcare professionals [12].

The utilization of personal protective equipment (PPE), such as masks, gloves, gowns, etc., is a fundamental cornerstone in the implementation of infection control measures within healthcare settings. This practice is crucial in safeguarding the well-being of both healthcare workers and patients. In the Netherlands, all healthcare facilities are adequately provisioned with the necessary PPEs to uphold the safety standards required for efficient healthcare delivery. However, Turkey faces challenges concerning the procurement and appropriate utilization of PPEs, as highlighted in previous studies [13–16]. The awareness and acceptance of respiratory masks, specifically FFP3 masks, by the majority of hospitals in Turkey were primarily instigated by the perceived threat of bird flu and subsequent recommendations from reputable organizations such as the CDC. At present, many Turkish hospitals are equipped with surgical and FFP3 masks, contrasting the situation in Dutch healthcare institutions where the more cost-effective FFP1 and FFP2 masks are predominantly utilized due to the lack of conclusive evidence mandating the use of FFP3 masks. The discomfort experienced by healthcare workers when wearing FFP3 masks, particularly those without a valve, is believed to contribute to a decrease in compliance with wearing them. Conversely, there have been reported cases of unnecessary extravagance in the procurement of certain PPEs, such as the improper use of gloves instead of following proper hand hygiene protocols and the excessive utilization of shoe covers in intensive care units (ICUs) and even by hospital visitors, leading to the inefficient allocation of limited resources. Despite the escalating challenges posed by nosocomial infections and the emergence of multidrug-resistant pathogens in Turkey, the national prioritization of infection control initiatives has historically been lacking. It wasn't until the 1980s, three decades after the establishment of infection control practices in the Netherlands, that Turkey began implementing infection control programs [17]. During this specific timeframe, a restricted quantity of medical facilities took the initiative to establish a nationwide monitoring system referred to as NOSO line. Following this, in the year 2006, the surveillance system underwent an expansion to include a multitude of medical centers under the supervision of the Refik Saydam Hygiene Center. At the present time, each and every medical institution in Turkey actively engages in submitting their infection rate data through this system and endeavors to improve infection control procedures based on the observations derived from these reports. Additionally, Turkey plays an active role as a member of the International Nosocomial Infection Control Consortium (INICC) [18], which is an international collaborative network committed to addressing healthcare-associated infections (HAIs) in countries with limited resources. Noteworthy is the establishment of the Turkish Society of Hospital Infection and Control in the year 2000, coupled with the development of infection control directives by the Ministry of Health in 2005, which indicate substantial advancements in reinforcing infection control measures in Turkey. Nonetheless, the structural framework for infection control, as demonstrated by the Dutch infection control center (WIP), had already been well-established long before these advancements, suggesting that healthcare professionals in Turkey are relatively new to the fundamentals of infection control strategies. Moreover, the delayed initiation of infection control initiatives in Turkey has led to a scarcity of infection control nurses in numerous medical centers, despite their crucial role in promoting effective infection control tactics. It was only recently that standardized educational programs for infection control nurses and physicians were introduced by the Ministry of Health in Turkey. Notably, neither Turkey nor the Netherlands have a dedicated medical specialty exclusively focused on infection control; rather, infection control teams in both nations are typically headed by medical microbiologists and experts in infectious diseases [19].

High rates of nosocomial infections in hospital environments create a significant motivator for healthcare providers, especially surgeons, to administer antibiotics that are unnecessary and not suitable, a behavior that has been widely observed. The comprehensive multicenter point-prevalence study conducted in Turkey uncovered that more than 50% of patients were prescribed antimicrobial medications in an inappropriate manner. Correspondingly, in a different investigation, a mere 26% of patients received the accurate antimicrobial prophylaxis. The inappropriate use of antimicrobials is expected to worsen the emergence of resistance among nosocomial pathogens. This issue is further complicated by the insufficient compliance with infection control protocols and the ineffectiveness of current infection control efforts, which results in the spread of these microorganisms within healthcare facilities. In the setting of Turkish university hospitals, the prevalence of methicillin-resistant *Staphylococcus aureus* (MRSA) and multidrug-resistant strains of *Acinetobacter* spp. is notably elevated, contributing to significant outbreaks.

Moreover, there is a growing incidence of Gram-negative bacteria producing extended-spectrum beta-lactamases (ESBLs) and vancomycin-resistant enterococci (VRE). Nonetheless, studies have shown that the adoption of a strong infection control strategy, like the "Search and Destroy" approach implemented in the Netherlands since 1986 following the emergence of MRSA, can effectively handle resistant strains. This approach highlights the early identification of carriers and the proactive isolation of patients upon admission as its fundamental principles. However, it is crucial to acknowledge that this strategy might present challenges in terms of resource allocation and financial burden, especially in areas with limited healthcare resources or high prevalence rates [20].

The utilization of molecular diagnostic techniques and typing methods to bolster infection control efforts is now a widely accepted norm in the majority of advanced healthcare systems globally. This paradigm shift signifies a pivotal advancement in the realm of healthcare, showcasing a commitment toward improving patient outcomes and reducing the spread of infectious diseases. Nevertheless, a glaring disparity exists in many Turkish university hospitals, where the absence of access to such sophisticated tools severely hampers their capacity to amass vital data essential for investigating outbreaks and devising prompt diagnostic remedies to fortify the containment of multidrug-resistant pathogens. This deficiency underscores a pressing need for urgent interventions to bridge the gap and equip these healthcare facilities with the necessary resources and technologies to effectively combat infectious diseases.

10.4 Summary

Fundamentally, the confluence of deficiencies in infrastructure, constraints in resources, complexities in human behavior, and the sluggish pace of establishing robust infection control protocols in specific low- and middle-income (LMI) nations present a formidable obstacle. The mitigation of these multifaceted challenges mandates a comprehensive approach tailored to the constrained-resource setting prevalent in these regions. Tackling the intricate interplay of these variables necessitates a nuanced and customized strategy that considers the distinctive circumstances and limitations characteristic of these countries. Consequently, efforts to enhance infection control measures in such settings must be underpinned by a thorough understanding of the local context and a commitment to fostering sustainable solutions that are both effective and contextually appropriate.

References

1. Raka L. Lowbury Lecture 2008: infection control and limited resources-searching for the best solutions. J Hosp Infect. 2009;72:292–8. https://doi.org/10.1016/j.jhin.2009.03.017.
2. Metan G, Alp E, Aygen B, Sumerkan B. Acinetobacter baumannii meningitis in post-neurosurgical patients: clinical outcome and impact of carbapenem resistance. J Antimicrob Chemother. 2007;60:197–9. https://doi.org/10.1093/jac/dkm181.

3. Metintas S, Akgun Y, Durmaz G, Kalyoncu C. Prevalence and characteristics of nosocomial infections in a Turkish university hospital. Am J Infect Control. 2004;32:409–13. https://doi.org/10.1016/j.ajic.2004.05.001.
4. Esen S, Leblebicioğlu H. Prevalence of nosocomial infections at intensive care units in Turkey: a multicentre 1-day point prevalence study. Scand J Infect Dis. 2004;36:144–8. https://doi.org/10.1080/00365540410019156.
5. PREZIES: Prevalentieonderzoek 2008. http://www.prezies.nl/zkh/prev/index.html.
6. Karabey S, Ay P, Derbentli S, Nakıpoğlu Y, Esen F. Handwashing frequencies in an intensive care unit. J Hosp Infect. 2002;50:36–41. https://doi.org/10.1053/jhin.2001.1132.
7. Sacar S, Turgut H, Kaleli I, Cevahir N, Asan A, Sacar M, Tekin K. Poor hospital infection control practice in hand hygiene, glove utilization, and usage of tourniquets. Am J Infect Control. 2006;34:606–9. https://doi.org/10.1016/j.ajic.2006.02.006.
8. Karabay O, Sencan I, Sahin I, Alpteker H, Ozcan A, Oksuz S. Compliance and efficacy of hand rubbing during in-hospital practice. Med Princ Pract. 2005;14:313–7. https://doi.org/10.1159/000086928.
9. Voss A, Widmer AF. No time for handwashing!? Hand washing versus alcoholic rub: can we afford 100% compliance? Infect Control Hosp Epidemiol. 1997;18:205–8. https://doi.org/10.1086/647590.
10. Alp E, Loefflen F, Doganay M, Voss A. Comparison of catheter care practices and catheter infection rates of Turkish and Dutch intensive care units in two university hospitals: a prospective study. Flora. 2009;14:153–8.
11. Yilmaz G, Caylan R, Aydin K, Topbas M, Koksal I. Effect of education on the rate of and the understanding of risk factors for intravascular catheter-related infections. Infect Control Hosp Epidemiol. 2007;28:689–94. https://doi.org/10.1086/517976.
12. Pittet D. The Lowbury lecture: behaviour in infection control. J Hosp Infect. 2004;58:1–13. https://doi.org/10.1016/j.jhin.2004.06.002.
13. Bijl D, Voss A. Infection control in the Netherlands. J Hosp Infect. 2001;47:169–72. https://doi.org/10.1053/jhin.2000.0885.
14. Leblebicioglu H, Unal S. The organization of hospital infection control in Turkey. J Hosp Infect. 2002;51:1–6. https://doi.org/10.1053/jhin.2002.1195.
15. Rosenthal VD, Maki DG, Graven N. The International Nosocomial Infection Control Consortium (INICC): goals and objectives, description of surveillance methods, and operational activities. Am J Infect Control. 2008;36:e1–e12.
16. Rosenthal VD. Device-associated nosocomial infections in limited-resources countries: findings of the International Nosocomial Infection Control Consortium (INICC). Am J Infect Control. 2008;36:S171.e7–e12. https://doi.org/10.1016/j.ajic.2008.10.009.
17. Usluer G, Ozgunes I, Leblebicioğlu H. A multicenter point-prevalence study: antimicrobial prescription frequencies in hospitalized patients in Turkey. Ann Clin Microbiol Antimicrob. 2005;4:16. https://doi.org/10.1186/1476-0711-4-16.
18. Bayram A, Balci I. Patterns of antimicrobial resistance in a surgical intensive care unit of a university hospital in Turkey. BMC Infect Dis. 2006;6:155. https://doi.org/10.1186/1471-2334-6-155.
19. Alp E, Esel D, Yildiz O, Voss A, Melchers W, Doganay M. Genotypic analysis of Acinetobacter bloodstream infection isolates in a Turkish university hospital. Scand J Infect Dis. 2006;38:335–40. https://doi.org/10.1080/00365540500488907.
20. Alp E, Klaassen CH, Doganay M, Altoprak U, Aydin K, Engin A, Kuzucu C, Ozinel MA, Turhan O, Voss A. MRSA genotypes in Turkey: persistence over 10 years of a single clone of ST239. J Infect. 2009;58:433–8. https://doi.org/10.1016/j.jinf.2009.04.006.

Chapter 11
Good Practices and Standard Operating Procedures for Sterilization Across Wards

11.1 Introduction

This scientific article focuses on the importance of sterilization and disinfection in hospital infection control activities. With numerous surgical and invasive procedures being performed daily in various healthcare facilities, there is a significant risk of introducing pathogens into patients' bodies through contact with medical devices and surgical instruments. Improperly sterilized or disinfected devices have been associated with a higher risk of transmitting infections such as hepatitis B virus (HBV), *Pseudomonas aeruginosa*, and *Acinetobacter* spp. The article emphasizes the need for adequate decontamination techniques for medical and surgical devices in all healthcare facilities to prevent outbreaks and infections [1]. This highlights the role of healthcare providers in reducing and eliminating such infections, emphasizing that every hospital should have its own guidelines for sterilizing and disinfecting items based on the intended use of medical devices and associated infections. Furthermore, the article discusses the increase in the frequency of newly emerging and multidrug-resistant pathogens in healthcare centers, for which few or no treatments are available. It underscores the importance of healthcare personnel, laboratory staff, and providers having a better understanding of sterilization and disinfection techniques to prevent the spread of these pathogens. Hence, it emphasizes the critical role of sterilization and disinfection in preventing the transmission of infections in healthcare settings. It calls for healthcare facilities to implement adequate decontamination techniques for medical and surgical devices and stresses the importance of healthcare providers having a comprehensive understanding of these techniques to prevent the spread of emerging and multidrug-resistant pathogens.

R. Chakraverty, A. K. Kundu, *Hospital-Acquired Infections in Intensive Care Unit and their Management*, https://doi.org/10.1007/978-981-96-0018-2_11

11.2 Cleaning

Before any reprocessing is conducted to achieve disinfection or sterility, it is imperative that all instruments and equipment undergo thorough cleaning. Failure to clean them adequately may result in the presence of organic matter, which can hinder the disinfectant or sterilant from making contact with the instrument. Additionally, this organic matter may potentially bind to and deactivate the chemical properties of the disinfectant. In cases where an instrument cannot be effectively cleaned, it becomes impossible to sterilize or disinfect it. Subsequent to the use of an instrument, it is recommended to wash it before proceeding with the drying process in order to eliminate any visible contamination. During this stage, the use of detergent or water is deemed suitable.

11.2.1 Manual Cleaning

All surfaces of the apparatus must be meticulously cleaned to ensure thorough reach of all channels and bores. When conducting manual washing of instruments, it is imperative to adhere to the subsequent protocols: don personal protective gear such as a plastic apron, thick rubber gloves, eye protection, a surgical mask, or a face shield [2].

1. Commence the procedure by clearing any observable residue on the device through a rinse in tepid water (15–18 °C).
2. Proceed to disassemble the instrument entirely and soak all components in warm water containing a biodegradable, noncorrosive, nonabrasive, low-foaming, and easily rinsed detergent.
3. Alternatively, utilize an enzymatic cleaner if deemed necessary. Ensure the complete removal of any apparent dirt from the instrument by strictly following the manufacturer's guidelines.
4. Conduct a final rinse in hot water, unless specifically advised against. Subsequently, dry the instrument either in a designated dry cabinet or manually with a clean, lint-free cloth. Conduct a thorough inspection to verify the cleanliness of the instrument.

11.2.2 Enzymatic Cleaners

Employed for the maintenance of fiber optic instruments, accessories, and other intricate items that present difficulties in terms of sanitation. It is essential to exercise caution while handling these products owing to their hazardous nature.

11.2.3 Ultrasonic Cleaners and Automated Washers [3]

Ultrasonic cleaners and automated washers are recommended for the cleaning of basic instruments that are capable of withstanding this particular process. The utilization of a machine to cleanse the instruments will significantly reduce the amount of manual handling required. It is imperative that these cleaning devices adhere to national regulations and standards and that they are operated in accordance with the guidelines provided by the manufacturer. It should be noted that ultrasonic cleaners do not serve as a method for disinfecting instruments. By generating high-frequency, high-energy soundwaves that impact the instrument/equipment, the debris is dislodged from the instrument or becomes more easily removable during the rinsing phase. However, these cleaning systems are unsuitable for cleaning cannulated instruments (as they are unable to reach the interior of the instrument), plastic materials, combinations of two or more different metals, as well as certain glass instruments, syringes, and lenses. Regular efficiency assessments should be conducted on a daily basis.

11.3 Disinfection

Disinfection is the process of eliminating microorganisms without achieving complete sterilization. It is commonly utilized to eradicate organisms found on delicate or heat-sensitive instruments that are unsuitable for sterilization or in cases where single-use items are unavailable. It is imperative to note that disinfection should not be considered a sterilization method and should not be employed as a convenient alternative to sterilization. Thermal disinfection, specifically, is unsuitable for instruments intended for critical applications as these instruments necessitate sterility. Various products and techniques offer diverse levels of disinfection, which are categorized as follows [4]:

(a) *High-level disinfection*: Eradicates all microorganisms with the exception of certain bacterial spores, particularly in instances of substantial contamination.
(b) *Intermediate disinfection*: Deactivates *Mycobacterium tuberculosis*, vegetative bacteria, most viruses, and the majority of fungi yet may not always eliminate bacterial spores.
(c) *Low-level disinfection*: Capable of eliminating most bacteria, certain viruses, and fungi but may not effectively target more resilient bacteria like *M. tuberculosis* or bacterial spores.

The two methodologies for disinfection encompass thermal disinfection and chemical disinfection. Thermal disinfection, applicable when the equipment's tolerance to heat and moisture processes is confirmed and sterilization is not necessary, proves to be an effective approach. The utilization of heat and water at a temperature that eradicates pathogenic, vegetative organisms stands out as a highly efficient disinfection technique. The efficacy of disinfection is contingent upon the water temperature and the duration of exposure of the instruments to said temperature. On the other hand, chemical disinfection's effectiveness is influenced by various factors including temperature, duration of contact, concentration, pH level, presence of organic or inorganic compounds, as well as the quantity and resilience of initial bio-microbials on the surface. Disinfectants for instruments are categorized into high, medium, or low levels, with compliance to manufacturer instructions determining the classification of disinfectants within these levels.

11.3.1 Selection of Disinfectants

In the realm of disinfection, the quest for a singular, perfect disinfectant remains elusive and perhaps unattainable. The diverse array of disinfectants available in the market cater to specific needs and purposes, thereby necessitating careful consideration during selection. Exclusive utilization of instrument-grade disinfectants is imperative when dealing with medical instruments and equipment, as they are specifically formulated for such delicate and critical applications. On the contrary, the deployment of hospital-grade or household-grade disinfectants on instruments is strictly contraindicated, as their efficacy is optimized for broader environmental sanitation purposes. Vigilant monitoring of the disinfectant solution is indispensable, particularly in scenarios where it serves multiple uses, to ensure its potency and effectiveness remain intact. Furthermore, adherence to proper storage protocols in alignment with manufacturers' guidelines is paramount to uphold the integrity of the disinfectant. Caution must be exercised to prevent any inadvertent contamination of the solution during dispensing for use, as even minor impurities can compromise its disinfecting capabilities.

Glutaraldehyde, being a chemical disinfectant, is generally considered the most suitable option for achieving a high level of disinfection in various settings. It is imperative that this particular chemical is utilized within a controlled environment that adheres to stringent safety protocols to ensure optimal effectiveness. Glutaraldehyde at a concentration of 2% has been identified as a suitable high-level disinfectant for a range of equipment such as endoscopes, respiratory therapy devices, and materials that are susceptible to damage from high temperatures. A minimum immersion duration of 20 min is recommended for achieving the desired disinfection outcomes. The delicate nature of flexible endoscopes makes them highly vulnerable to damage and presents challenges in terms of effective disinfection procedures. Hence, it is of utmost significance to emphasize the crucial step of thorough mechanical cleansing prior to the initiation of any sterilization or disinfection processes.

11.4 Sterilization

The definitions and standards for sterilization, disinfection, and cleaning as defined by the Clinical and Laboratory Standards Institute and the International Organization of Standardization. Sterilization is defined as the complete elimination or destruction of all forms of microbial life, including both vegetative and spore forms, achieved through various physical and chemical methods. Chemical sterilants, such as peracetic acid, glutaraldehyde, ortho-phthalaldehyde, and hydrogen peroxide, are used for longer durations to destroy all forms of microbes. Disinfection, on the other hand, involves the complete elimination of vegetative forms of microorganisms, excluding bacterial spores, from inanimate objects. High-level disinfectants, such as glutaraldehyde, ortho-phthalaldehyde, hydrogen peroxide, hypochlorite, and hypochlorous acid, are capable of killing a high number of microorganisms except spores, while intermediate and low-level disinfectants act against specific types of microorganisms and are used for specific items. Decontamination and cleaning are processes that remove pathogenic microorganisms from objects and visible soil from surfaces and objects, respectively. Antisepsis involves the removal of germs from the skin, either for the patient's skin (disinfection of living tissue) or the healthcare worker's skin (reduction or removal of transient microbes). Germicides, including antiseptics and disinfectants, are classified based on the type of microorganism they target, such as virucides, fungicides, bactericides, sporicides, and tuberculocides. This underscores the importance of understanding the distinctions between these terms and the specific methods and agents that are used for sterilization, disinfection, and cleaning. It outlines the technical definitions and criteria for each process and provides a comprehensive overview of the different types of chemicals and methods employed in these practices. Invasive medical procedures pose a significant risk of introducing pathogenic microbes to patients, leading to infections if proper disinfection or sterilization of reusable medical equipment is not performed. The level of disinfection or sterilization required depends on the intended use of the object, with critical, semicritical, and noncritical items necessitating sterilization, high-level disinfection, and low-level disinfection, respectively. It is essential that cleaning precedes high-level disinfection and sterilization. Users need to carefully consider the advantages and disadvantages of specific methods when choosing a disinfection or sterilization process. Adhering to these recommendations is crucial for improving disinfection and sterilization practices in healthcare facilities and subsequently reducing infections associated with contaminated patient-care items.

Almost half a century ago, precisely 50 years in the past, Earle H. Spaulding developed a systematic and rational approach to the crucial processes of disinfection and sterilization when dealing with patient-care items and equipment within healthcare settings. This classification system introduced by Spaulding has proven to be exceptionally lucid and coherent, to the extent that it has been preserved, enhanced, and effectively applied by professionals in infection control and other relevant stakeholders when strategizing techniques for disinfection or sterilization procedures [5]. Spaulding's conceptualization revolved around the notion that the comprehension of disinfection processes could be significantly facilitated by categorizing instruments and materials used for patient care into three distinct groups based on the level of infection risk associated with their utilization. The three specific categories delineated by Spaulding encompass critical, semicritical, and noncritical items. Notably, these terms are expressly employed in the Centers for Disease Control and Prevention's (CDC) authoritative documents such as the "Guidelines for Environmental Infection Control in Healthcare Facilities" and the "Guideline for Disinfection and Sterilization in Healthcare Facilities." These categories are pivotal in delineating the protocols and techniques required to achieve sterilization, high-level disinfection, and low-level disinfection in healthcare settings [6]. Despite the enduring relevance of this classification system, there exist instances of disinfection studies involving challenging microorganisms such as prions, viruses, and other microorganisms that pose a significant challenge to the prevailing definitions and anticipated outcomes of high-level disinfection (HLD) and low-level disinfection [7, 8].

Sterilization [9], which refers to the eradication of all microorganisms, can be accomplished through various methods, either physical or chemical in nature. The necessity of sterilization becomes evident when dealing with medical devices that are intended to penetrate sterile body sites. It is crucial to emphasize the initial step of cleaning to eliminate any visible soiling present in reusable equipment before proceeding with the sterilization process. Moreover, it is imperative to designate only those materials that have been properly wrapped or packed as sterile. Prior to subjecting any instrument or equipment to steam sterilization, a series of checks must be conducted to ensure the effectiveness of the process. Firstly, it is essential to ascertain that the instrument is capable of withstanding the sterilization procedure. Secondly, adequate cleaning of the instrument must be confirmed. Additionally, any special treatment requirements for the instrument should be identified. Lastly, meticulous records regarding the sterilization process and the traceability of instruments must be diligently maintained. The various methods of sterilization outlined below are specifically formulated to provide a sterility assurance level of at least one in a million, denoted as 10^{-6}, as long as the process is duly validated and aligns with the manufacturer's stipulated guidelines. Notably, equipment such as ultraviolet light units, incubators, microwave ovens, and domestic ovens are deemed unsuitable for sterilization purposes.

11.4.1 Moist Sterilization (Steam Under Pressure)

One of the most efficient and reliable methods of sterilization is steam under pressure, also known as moist heat sterilization. This method stands out for its ability to achieve sterility in instruments and equipment while simultaneously ensuring the sterilization and drying of sterile packages within the cycle. Particularly recommended for office-based practices, various types of steam-under-pressure sterilizers, commonly referred to as autoclaves, exist. Downward displacement sterilizers, available in jacketed or non-jacketed forms, are specifically designed for the sterilization of waste, solutions, and instruments. On the other hand, self-contained benchtop sterilizers are highly favored in office-based settings due to their capacity to process small quantities or relatively straightforward items. It is worth noting that benchtop sterilizers do not accommodate wrapped items, necessitating immediate use of items post-sterilization. Furthermore, prevacuum sterilizers, optimized for the sterilization of clean instruments, gowns, drapes, toweling, and other dry materials essential for surgical procedures, are not suitable for liquid sterilization. These sterilizers are tailored to meet the specific requirements of surgical settings, ensuring the maintenance of a sterile environment conducive to successful medical interventions.

11.4.2 Dry Heat Sterilization [10]

Dry heat sterilization is a method of sterilization that involves the use of hot air to eliminate pathogens through the process of oxidation. The effectiveness of dry heat sterilization has been limited due to the challenges associated with maintaining a consistent temperature throughout the entire sterilization process. Furthermore, the high temperatures and extended duration required to achieve sterility make this method less than ideal for many applications. It is crucial to adhere to the instructions provided by the manufacturers and to refrain from opening the unit's door while it is in the midst of the sterilizing cycle.

11.4.3 Ethylene Oxide

Ethylene oxide (EO) gas, which is commonly known as ethylene oxide, is deemed suitable for the sterilization of medical instruments and equipment manufactured from materials sensitive to heat or those containing delicate electronic components. The duration necessary for the completion of the sterilization process is contingent upon factors such as temperature variations, humidity levels, and the concentration of the gas utilized. It is imperative that the gas effectively permeates the packaging material and reaches every nook and cranny of the instrument or equipment in need of sterilization. The timeframe allocated for this intricate process typically ranges from a minimum of 12 h to sometimes exceeding a duration of more than 24 h. Due to the inherent toxicity associated with ethylene oxide, stringent regulations are in place within healthcare facilities to govern its usage, ensuring the utmost safety of the personnel involved. Adherence to meticulous guidelines is crucial to mitigate any potential risks. Moreover, it is essential to strictly adhere to the instructions provided by the manufacturer concerning the packaging protocols, sterilization procedures, validation processes, and post-sterilization aeration steps.

11.4.4 Low-Temperature Sterilization

Automated chemical systems utilizing low-temperature techniques, such as hydrogen peroxide plasma, operate within a fully automated cycle that is capable of achieving low-temperature sterilization with minimal moisture content in a timeframe ranging from 45 to 80 min, which is contingent upon the specific model of sterilizer utilized for the process. It is imperative that the packaging employed in this method consists of nonwoven/non-cellulose polypropylene wraps to ensure the efficacy of the sterilization procedure. Another method for achieving sterilization at low temperatures is through the utilization of peracetic acid, whereby a concentration of 0.2% of this chemical is placed within an environmentally sealed chamber that operates as part of a fully automated processing system. Through this method, the sterilization process is able to attain a state of moist, low-temperature sterilization within a time frame of 25–30 min.

11.4.5 Gamma Radiation

In certain cases, Gamma radiation can be utilized for irradiation purposes and is offered by select commercial gamma irradiation facilities. However, it is important to note that this method is not readily accessible for implementation within healthcare facilities. It is crucial to understand that only instruments and equipment that have undergone the complete sterilizing process can be deemed as truly sterile. To achieve sterility, items must be appropriately wrapped or packaged in a manner that meets the necessary standards. Various materials can be employed for packaging purposes, including paper, which serves the purpose of preventing contamination as long as its integrity remains intact. Furthermore, paper has the ability to maintain sterility over an extended period, can function as a sterile field, and can also be utilized for wrapping devices that are soiled post-procedure. Additionally, nonwoven disposable textiles and containers can be utilized for packaging, with the caveat that containers should only be used if they are designated for a single treatment procedure for a singular patient. Prior to usage, it is the responsibility of the end-user to conduct a thorough check of the physical integrity of the package to ensure its effectiveness.

Quality control parameters for the sterilization process, which also function as a checklist for the sterilization department, encompass various essential elements such as load number, load content, temperature and time exposure record chart, physical/chemical testing, and biological testing utilizing *Bacillus subtilis*. It is imperative to conduct and meticulously document regular engineering maintenance on sterilization equipment to ensure optimal functionality. It is advised against boiling medical devices for reuse due to the inability to guarantee sterility. Yet, in specific resource-constrained scenarios where steam sterilization is unfeasible, it is recommended to meticulously clean these items and subject them to a cycle in a pressure cooker lasting 30 min.

11.5 Environmental Management Measures [11]

Environmental management measures are crucial in the context of preventing hospital-associated infections (HAI), with a particular emphasis on the significance of maintaining a hygienic environment. Numerous factors come into play, encompassing the layout of patient care areas, operating rooms, air quality, water supply, and laundry, all of which can significantly impact the transmission of HAI.

11.6 Management of Cleanliness in Premises/Buildings [12]

When it comes to premises/buildings, meticulous facility design and planning are paramount to ensure optimal conditions. This includes provisions for an adequate safe water supply, implementation of appropriate cleaning practices, allocation of sufficient floor space for beds, provision of adequate interbed space, availability of ample hand washing facilities, establishment of proper ventilation in isolation rooms and high-risk areas such as operation theatres, transplant units, and intensive care areas. Additionally, there should be adequate isolation facilities catering to airborne, droplet, contact isolation, and protective environments. Furthermore, measures should be in place to regulate traffic flow to minimize exposure of high-risk patients and facilitate patient transport, as well as precautions to prevent patient exposure to fungal spores during renovation activities. It is also essential to implement strategies to control rodents, pests, and other vectors, in addition to ensuring appropriate waste management facilities and practices are in place.

11.7 Air

Ventilation systems must be meticulously designed and upheld to reduce microbial contamination. Regular cleaning of air conditioning filters is essential, and caution should be exercised in high-risk areas to avoid fans that could disseminate airborne pathogens. Special ventilation systems are imperative for high-risk zones like operating rooms, critical care units, and transplant units. In high-risk areas, filtration systems (air handling units) ought to be equipped with high-efficiency particulate air (HEPA) filters. Hospital constructions should incorporate unidirectional laminar airflow systems in appropriate areas. Ultraclean air is particularly beneficial in certain surgical settings such as cardiac surgery, neurosurgery, implant surgery theatres, and transplant units. Critical parameters for air quality in the operating room encompass the frequent maintenance and validation of filter efficacy as per the manufacturer's guidelines, monitoring the pressure gradient across the filter bed and in the operation theatre, ensuring a minimum of 15 air changes per hour, maintaining a temperature between 20 and 22 °C, and controlling humidity between 30 and

60% to impede bacterial proliferation. Furthermore, adequate ventilation is crucial for general areas lacking air conditioning.

11.8 Special Air Handling for Airborne Precautions

In order to maintain a safe and healthy environment in contaminated areas, it is highly recommended to implement a system that creates negative air pressure, which should be vented to the external atmosphere. Additionally, this approach is essential for effectively isolating patients who are suffering from infections that are known to spread through the airborne route. It is advised that an air-handling system be put in place, capable of providing a frequency of 6–12 air changes per hour while ensuring that the air is being expelled outside after passing through a filtration mechanism, thereby reducing the risk of contamination.

To guarantee the efficacy of these systems, it is imperative that they undergo thorough inspections conducted by expert engineering services to verify that the rooms are indeed operating under negative pressure conditions as intended. For healthcare facilities that lack designated "negative pressure" rooms, viable alternatives include utilizing an air-conditioned single room equipped with an exhaust system or opting for a well-ventilated room to meet the necessary requirements for infection control. In instances where an air-conditioned single room is not feasible, especially in resource-constrained settings, a practical solution would be to strategically place a fan within the room to facilitate the direction of airflow towards an open window leading outside.

Moreover, it is crucial to emphasize the importance of maintaining the integrity of the isolation area by ensuring that the door or doors leading to adjacent areas or corridors are securely shut at all times to prevent the potential spread of contaminants. By adhering to these recommendations and guidelines, healthcare facilities can effectively mitigate the risk of airborne infections and create a safer environment for both patients and healthcare workers alike.

11.9 Protective Environment [13]

A necessity for a protective environment might be deemed necessary for certain patients who are experiencing neutropenia, a condition characterized by a low count of neutrophils in the blood, which can significantly compromise the immune system. The requirement for ultraclean unidirectional air is particularly crucial in specialized units like hematology or intensive care, owing to the heightened level of immunosuppression observed in the patient population being treated within these settings. In order to effectively reduce the presence of airborne particles within these environments, it is imperative that the air circulation system is designed to push air into the room at a minimum velocity of 0.25 m/s, a requirement that can be met by utilizing high-efficiency particulate air (HEPA) filters. These filters are specifically engineered to trap and remove particles of a certain size, ensuring that the air entering the room undergoes thorough purification. For instance, if 77 particles measuring 0.3 μm in diameter are successfully eliminated by the HEPA filter, the air quality within the room can be classified as pristine, devoid of any bacterial contamination that could pose a risk to the vulnerable patients under care.

Moreover, there are additional crucial measures that must be implemented to safeguard patients with severely compromised immune systems, including but not limited to the following protocols:

- Healthcare workers and visitors must exercise utmost caution and avoid direct contact with the patient if they are exhibiting any signs of infection, such as symptoms associated with upper respiratory tract infections or visible lesions like herpes simplex blisters.
- In situations where deemed necessary, both staff members and visitors entering the premises should adhere to strict guidelines regarding the utilization of personal protective equipment, thereby creating an additional barrier of defense against potential microorganism transmission to the patient.
- It is advisable to refrain from placing flowers or plants in the patient's room, as these natural elements can harbor various pathogens that may pose a threat to the patient's delicate health condition.
- Maintaining a clean and organized environment is paramount, as clutter and untidiness can serve as breeding grounds for harmful microorganisms, thereby increasing the risk of infection transmission.
- Routine environmental cleaning practices must be rigorously carried out at least twice daily, with a focus on utilizing damp dusting techniques exclusively to prevent the generation of aerosols that could inadvertently spread contaminants.
- During all clinical procedures, strict adherence to aseptic techniques is nonnegotiable, as any breaches in sterile protocols could potentially introduce harmful pathogens and compromise the patients already compromised immune defenses.

11.10 Water

The provision of safe water within healthcare facilities is of paramount importance to ensure the well-being of patients and staff. It is imperative that any water storage tanks present within the facility undergo regular and thorough cleaning procedures to mitigate the risk of waterborne infections. Moreover, periodic sampling of the water should be conducted to assess its quality and detect any potential bacterial contamination that may compromise the safety of the water supply.

11.11 Safe Drinking Water

In instances where safe water is not readily available, one recommended method is to boil the water for a duration of 5 min as a means of disinfection. Alternatively, the utilization of water purification units can also serve as an effective measure to ensure the provision of safe and potable water. Furthermore, it is crucial that water is stored in a hygienic environment to prevent any form of contamination. Strict protocols should be in place to prohibit the entry of hands into the water storage containers in order to maintain the integrity of the water supply. To facilitate the dispensing of water from storage containers, it is advisable to utilize outlets equipped with closure devices or taps to minimize the risk of external contamination. Additionally, regular cleaning of the storage containers and water coolers is essential to uphold the quality and safety of the water stored within the facility. Adherence to these meticulous practices is vital to safeguard the health and well-being of all individuals who rely on the healthcare facility for their water needs.

11.12 Hospital Environment Cleaning

Routine cleaning plays a crucial role in maintaining a hygienic and dust-free environment within hospital facilities, ensuring the overall safety of patients and staff. The presence of numerous micro-organisms within visible dirt underscores the significance of regular cleaning practices in the elimination of such contaminants. It is notable that administrative and office spaces devoid of direct patient contact necessitate conventional domestic cleaning methods. Conversely, areas dedicated to patient care demand a more thorough approach, typically involving wet mopping as opposed to dry sweeping, which is discouraged due to its limited effectiveness. The utilization of a neutral detergent solution emerges as a key factor in enhancing the efficacy of cleaning procedures, contributing to a higher standard of cleanliness.

11.13 Conclusion

In this regard, the application of hot water at a temperature of 80 °C proves to be a valuable and efficient environmental cleaning agent. However, it is generally advised against conducting bacteriological testing of the environment unless there is a specific need to investigate a potential source of an outbreak. Immediate attention is required for areas visibly contaminated with blood or bodily fluids, necessitating a prompt cleaning regimen using detergent and water. Special precautions are warranted for isolation rooms and spaces accommodating patients with confirmed transmissible infectious diseases, mandating a daily cleaning routine with a detergent/disinfectant solution. Furthermore, the daily cleaning of all horizontal surfaces and toilet areas is essential to uphold high standards of hygiene within healthcare settings. Surfaces can be categorized into two distinct groups based on their level of hand contact, with floors and ceilings falling under the category of minimal hand contact surfaces, while surfaces subject to frequent skin contact are classified as "frequently touched" or "high risk" surfaces. The determination of cleaning methods, frequency, and products utilized is contingent upon a thorough risk analysis, in alignment with the established policies of healthcare facilities. Notably, frequently touched surfaces in patient care zones require diligent cleaning using a detergent solution, and they should be cleaned more frequently compared to surfaces with minimal hand contact. In the realm of infection control, professionals typically adopt a risk-assessment approach to identify frequently touched surfaces, subsequently devising a comprehensive cleaning strategy and schedule in collaboration with the housekeeping staff. In cases where multidrug-resistant organisms (MDROs) are suspected or confirmed to be present, an intensified approach to routine cleaning is imperative. This involves the sequential use of a detergent solution followed by a disinfectant to ensure that surfaces are effectively cleaned and disinfected, thereby mitigating the risk of transmission.

References

1. Centers for Disease Control and Prevention. National hospital discharge survey: 2010 table, procedures by selected patient characteristics-number by procedure category and age; 2010.
2. CDC. Updated guidelines for evaluating public health surveillance systems: recommendations from the Guidelines Working Group. MMWR. 2001;50:1–51.
3. CDC. Workbook for designing, implementing and evaluating a sharps injury prevention program; 2009. http://www.cdc.gov/sharpssafety/.
4. Chandy SJ, Michael JS, Veeraraghavan B, Abraham OC, Bachhav SS, Kshirsagar NA. ICMR programme on Antibiotic Stewardship, Prevention of Infection & Control (ASPIC). Indian J Med Res. 2014;139:226–30.
5. Peery AF, Dellon ES, Lund J. Burden of gastrointestinal disease in the United States: 2012 update. Gastroenterology. 2012;143:1179–87.
6. Epstein L, Hunter JC, Arwady MA. New Delhi metallo-beta-lactamase-producing carbapenem-resistant Escherichia coli associated with exposure to duodenoscopes. JAMA. 2014;312:1447–55.
7. Wendorf KA, Kay M, Baliga C. Endoscopic retrograde cholangiopancreatography-associated AmpC *Escherichia coli* outbreak. Infect Control Hosp Epidemiol. 2015;36:634–42.
8. Rutala WA, Weber DJ. Disinfection and sterilization of prion-contaminated medical instruments, reply to Belay. Infect Control Hosp Epidemiol. 2010;31:1306–7.
9. Dharan S, Pittet D. Environmental controls in operating theatres. J Hosp Infect. 2002;51:79–84.
10. Gaind R, Deb M. Infection control policy. New Delhi: Vardhaman Mahavir Medical College & Safdarjung Hospital; 2010.
11. Grayson ML, Russo PL. The national hand hygiene initiative. Med J Aust. 2009;191(8):420–1.
12. HPS. Standard infection control precautions—literature review: control of the environment. Health Protection Scotland, National Health Service Scotland; 2006.
13. ICMR. Infection control assessment tool. New Delhi: ICMR; 2015.

Chapter 12
Future Directions and the Way Ahead

12.1 Introduction

Historically, the field of infection prevention and control (IPC) has conventionally provided a systematic and unbiased method for identifying infections and infectious risks among both patients and healthcare workers. The year 1986 marked the beginning of the first-ever "Infection Control Week," a time when the majority of acute healthcare services were primarily delivered in hospital settings. While hospitals in that era did integrate "prevention" into their IPC programs, their main emphasis was on surveillance activities, with a considerable portion of resources dedicated to this aspect. Throughout the 1980s, healthcare services involving invasive procedures or medical devices were mainly conducted in acute care facilities. Detailed information regarding rates of healthcare-associated infections (HAIs) [1, 2] was not shared with external parties or individuals outside the hospital premises. Furthermore, at that time, responsibilities related to IPC were typically carried out by appointed infection control practitioners (ICPs) rather than by interdisciplinary teams. It was during this period that the notion of bioterrorism was mostly seen in the realm of science fiction, AIDS emerged as a significant disease, methicillin-resistant *Staphylococcus aureus* began moving from academic tertiary care centers to mainstream community hospitals, and healthcare professionals were enhancing their expertise through insights drawn from specialized areas of study.

The transformation within the healthcare landscape was characterized by a shift away from traditional structures and practices that were designed for organizations with well-defined knowledge domains toward the adoption of processes suitable for a complex adaptive system. This shift in focus necessitated the integration and interaction of services and departments that were previously built on disparate knowledge bases. The newer framework emphasized the importance of performance enhancement and required the implementation of cost-cutting measures. By the year 2009, complex healthcare procedures and technologies were no longer limited

R. Chakraverty, A. K. Kundu, *Hospital-Acquired Infections in Intensive Care Unit and their Management*, https://doi.org/10.1007/978-981-96-0018-2_12

to acute care facilities but had spread to various settings such as long-term care facilities, ambulatory care centers, and even patient residences. Discussions were also underway regarding providing postoperative care at facilities near surgical centers. Infection preventionists (IPs) encountered challenges in establishing infection prevention and control (IPC) programs in these emerging environments due to a lack of substantial evidence to support their recommendations.

Many non-acute care settings did not have clear infection criteria, neglected to investigate infections thoroughly, relied on empirical antibiotic practices, and lacked standardized measurement denominators. IPC personnel were also responsible for developing strategies to address evolving biological threats like multidrug-resistant organisms, severe acute respiratory syndrome, and infectious diseases such as pandemic influenza. IPs took a leading role in implementing intervention bundles that, when combined with the efforts of other healthcare professionals, led to significant improvements in outcomes for patients requiring central vascular lines or ventilator support. Furthermore, current perspectives highlight the importance of recognizing that although healthcare procedures and devices have become more complex and technologically advanced, fundamental principles remain crucial [3, 4]. It is now widely acknowledged that isolated actions within healthcare systems can have far-reaching consequences across various processes and components. Success in achieving positive outcomes is dependent on the synergistic interaction of different aspects of care, including mechanical-physical, psychological, social, emotional, and spiritual dimensions. The evolving healthcare environment demands a holistic approach that considers the interconnectedness of these different facets to ensure optimal patient outcomes. This recognition underscores the critical role played by healthcare professionals in adapting to the changing landscape and embracing a comprehensive approach to patient care that addresses a wide range of needs and challenges [5].

As IPs look toward the future, they may need to consider potential changes that could impact the healthcare landscape. These changes might involve the utilization of antiaging medications to address the needs of an aging population, a potential increase in the prevalence of chronic illnesses due to various factors such as lifestyle changes and environmental issues, the automation of language translation through the use of advanced machine learning technologies to improve communication with diverse patient populations. Additionally, there could be a shift toward the adoption of universal electronic medical records that are carried by all patients to ensure seamless information sharing among healthcare providers, innovative techniques for drug delivery to enhance treatment outcomes, surveillance systems conducted via electronic means to monitor and prevent infectious disease outbreaks, an increase in xenotransplantation for patients in need of organ transplants, the availability of geographic information systems for tracking the movements of patients and healthcare personnel to improve resource allocation and response times, and a potential decrease in reimbursement for healthcare services, which could impact the delivery of care and resource allocation in healthcare settings.

In the current landscape, healthcare systems in the United States and other countries are facing complex challenges in reform efforts. Within the field of infection prevention and control (IPC), there are important questions that need to be addressed regarding the potential impact of proposed healthcare reforms on infection risks. It is crucial to understand how new healthcare systems can help mitigate infection risks, whether certain patient demographics may face increased infection risks due to healthcare changes, and how IPC practices will influence patient safety within evolving healthcare frameworks.

By the year 2009, the role of the infection preventionist (IP) had evolved significantly from being primarily focused on data collection and infection control advice to taking on a more proactive leadership role in healthcare improvement initiatives. IPs are now involved in making decisions related to resource allocation for evidence-based infection control practices, demonstrating a shift toward a more strategic and impactful role within healthcare settings. The field of IPC has advanced since 1986, requiring IPs to expand their expertise beyond traditional areas such as microbiology, epidemiology, and infectious diseases. IPs now need to acquire knowledge in emerging areas such as human factors engineering, data analytics, healthcare economics, and biomedical ethics to effectively navigate the complex healthcare landscape.

Recent and expected changes necessitate infection preventionists (IPs) to closely examine the impact of modifications in infection prevention and control (IPC) practices on patient outcomes. The heightened focus on accountability and transparency within the public healthcare-associated infections (HAI) reporting system raises the question of whether it has effectively improved patient outcomes. Additionally, the implementation of electronic health records and sophisticated data analysis systems prompts an inquiry into their contribution to enhancing patient care. IPs must now consider how they will actively participate in discussions regarding the cost-benefit analyses of various infection prevention technologies. Furthermore, as healthcare systems become more complex, IPs need to contemplate their roles in environments where patients with sufficient resources can access advanced infection prevention tools or procedures to further enhance safety measures. It is imperative to analyze the evolving landscape of healthcare and the factors that will shape its future. The contemporary issues surrounding infection prevention and control in healthcare are closely linked to events like the International Infection Control Week, highlighting their significance on a global scale. While we believe that the work of IPs is crucial to the healthcare sector, it is essential to ascertain whether policymakers and regulators share this perspective. To predict how IPC will be incorporated into future healthcare systems, active involvement in decision-making processes by individuals and organizations is the most viable approach. This proactive engagement will be instrumental in shaping new healthcare systems or restructuring existing ones for the betterment of patient care and overall public health [6].

12.2 Summary

Our involvement in low- and middle-income countries (LMICs) is focused on highlighting the unique contributions of infection prevention within the healthcare sector, with the objective of increasing its recognition and establishing a platform for clarifying the importance of infection prevention and control (IPC) practices for both healthcare providers and the wider communities they serve. Organizations such as APIC, the Society for Healthcare Epidemiology of America, and various governmental bodies at global, national, regional, state, and local levels, in addition to infection preventionists (IPs), have the opportunity to utilize the International Infection Prevention week as a moment for reflection on these critical issues and to emphasize the essential role of IPC in safeguarding patient well-being. Participating in proactive dialogues and initiatives related to these aforementioned concerns is positioned to seamlessly embed the crucial and irreplaceable component of IPC into the complex framework of national and global healthcare systems. Through fostering conversations and initiatives that tackle these challenges, we are essentially weaving the significant and indispensable function of IPC into the broader scope of national and global healthcare, ultimately improving patient safety and healthcare outcomes.

References

1. Association Professionals in Infection Control and Epidemiology. International infection prevention week. http://www.apic.org/AM/Template.cfm?Section=2009_International_Infection_Prevention_Week&Template. Accessed 31 Aug 2009.
2. National Infection Control Week, Community and Hospital Infection Control Organization-Canada (CHICA) news and features. http://www.chica.org/news_icweek.html. Accessed 31 Aug 2009.
3. Building the infection prevention system of tomorrow: proceedings of the 2007 APIC Futures Summit. Am J Infect Control. 2008;36:232–40.
4. The fifth evolutionary era in infection control: interventional epidemiology. Am J Infect Control. 2000;28:30–43.
5. The infection control community's response to the agenda for change. Am J Infect Control. 1989;17:241–3.
6. Who is steering the ship? External influences on infection control programs. Clin Infect Dis. 2008;46:1746–50.

GPSR Compliance

The European Union's (EU) General Product Safety Regulation (GPSR) is a set of rules that requires consumer products to be safe and our obligations to ensure this.

If you have any concerns about our products, you can contact us on ProductSafety@springernature.com

In case Publisher is established outside the EU, the EU authorized representative is:

Springer Nature Customer Service Center GmbH
Europaplatz 3
69115 Heidelberg, Germany

Batch number: 10732044

Printed by Printforce, the Netherlands